OrthoBiologics in Sports Medicine

Editors

BRIAN J. COLE
RACHEL M. FRANK

CLINICS IN SPORTS MEDICINE

www.sportsmed.theclinics.com

Consulting Editor
MARK D. MILLER

January 2019 • Volume 38 • Number 1

ELSEVIER

1600 John F. Kennedy Boulevard • Suite 1800 • Philadelphia, Pennsylvania, 19103-2899

http://www.theclinics.com

CLINICS IN SPORTS MEDICINE Volume 38, Number 1
January 2019 ISSN 0278-5919, ISBN-13: 978-0-323-65494-4

Editor: Lauren Boyle
Developmental Editor: Donald Mumford

Clinics in Sports Medicine (ISSN 0278-5919) is published quarterly by Elsevier Inc., 360 Park Avenue South, New York, NY 10010-1710. Months of issue are January, April, July, and October. Business and Editorial Offices: 1600 John F. Kennedy Blvd., Ste. 1800, Philadelphia, PA 19103-2899. Customer Service Office: 3251 Riverport Lane, Maryland Heights, MO 63043. Periodicals postage paid at New York, NY and additional mailing offices. Subscription prices are $364.00 per year (US individuals), $698.00 per year (US institutions), $100.00 per year (US students), $405.00 per year (Canadian individuals), $861.00 per year (Canadian institutions), $235.00 (Canadian students), $475.00 per year (foreign individuals), $861.00 per year (foreign institutions), and $235.00 per year (foreign students). Foreign air speed delivery is included in all *Clinics* subscription prices. All prices are subject to change without notice. **POSTMASTER:** Send address changes to *Clinics in Sports Medicine*, Elsevier Health Sciences Division, Subscription Customer Service, 3251 Riverport Lane, Maryland Heights, MO 63043. Customer Service (orders, claims, online, change of address): Elsevier Health Sciences Division, Subscription Customer Service, 3251 Riverport Lane, Maryland Heights, MO 63043. **Tel: 1-800-654-2452 (U.S. and Canada); 314-447-8871 (outside U.S. and Canada). Fax: 314-447-8029. E-mail: journalscustomerservice-usa@elsevier.com (for print support); journalsonlinesupport-usa@elsevier.com (for online support).**

Reprints. For copies of 100 or more of articles in this publication, please contact the Commercial Reprints Department, Elsevier Inc., 360 Park Avenue South, New York, NY 10010-1710. Tel.: 212-633-3874; Fax: 212-633-3820; E-mail: reprints@elsevier.com.

Clinics in Sports Medicine is covered in *MEDLINE/PubMed (Index Medicus) Current Contents/Clinical Medicine, Excerpta Medica,* and *ISI/Biomed.*

Contributors

CONSULTING EDITOR

MARK D. MILLER, MD
S. Ward Casscells Professor, Head, Department of Orthopaedic Surgery, Division of Sports Medicine, University of Virginia, Charlottesville, Virginia; Team Physician, Miller Review Course, Harrisonburg, Virginia

EDITORS

BRIAN J. COLE, MD, MBA
Associate Chairman and Professor, Department of Orthopedics, Chairman, Department of Surgery, Rush OPH, Managing Partner, Midwest Orthopaedics at Rush, Sports Medicine and Surgery, Shoulder, Elbow, and Knee Care, Section Head, Cartilage Restoration Center at Rush, Team Physician, Chicago Bulls and Chicago White Sox, Rush University Medical Center, Chicago, Illinois

RACHEL M. FRANK, MD
Assistant Professor, Sports Medicine and Shoulder Surgery, Assistant Professor, Department of Orthopaedic Surgery, University of Colorado School of Medicine, Aurora, Colorado

AUTHORS

JAKOB ACKERMANN, MD
Orthopedic Research Fellow, Department of Orthopedic Surgery, Brigham and Women's Hospital, Boston, Massachusetts

ZACH S. AMAN, BA
Biomedical Engineering Researcher, Steadman Philippon Research Institute, Vail, Colorado

ADAM ANZ, MD
Attending Surgeon, Andrews Institute, Andrews Research and Education Foundation, Gulf Breeze, Florida

JACOB G. CALCEI, MD
Orthopaedic Surgery Resident, Department of Sports Medicine and Shoulder, Hospital for Special Surgery, New York, New York

JORGE CHAHLA, MD, PhD
Orthopaedic Surgery Sports Medicine Fellow, Midwest Orthopaedics at Rush, Chicago, Illinois

KEVIN CHRISTENSEN, MD
Orthopedic Sports Medicine Fellow, Andrews Institute, Gulf Breeze, Florida

BRIAN J. COLE, MD, MBA
Associate Chairman and Professor, Department of Orthopedics, Chairman, Department of Surgery, Rush OPH, Managing Partner, Midwest Orthopaedics at Rush, Sports Medicine and Surgery, Shoulder, Elbow, and Knee Care, Section Head, Cartilage Restoration Center at Rush, Team Physician, Chicago Bulls and Chicago White Sox, Rush University Medical Center, Chicago, Illinois

BENJAMIN COX, DO
Director of Regenerative Medicine, Central Michigan University, Orthopedic Sports Medicine Fellow, Andrews Institute, Gulf Breeze, Florida

ALESSANDRO D'ANGELO, MD
Department of Orthopaedic, Traumatology and Rehabilitation, Azienda Ospedaliero Universitaria Città della Salute e della Scienza, CTO Hospital, Turin, Italy

MALCOLM R. DeBAUN, MD
Department of Orthopedic Surgery, Stanford University, Redwood City, California

BERARDO DI MATTEO, MD
Department of Biomedical Sciences, Humanitas University, Humanitas Clinical and Research Center, Rozzano, Milan, Italy

JASON L. DRAGOO, MD
Department of Orthopedic Surgery, Stanford University, Redwood City, California

ROBERT A. DUERR, MD
Assistant Professor of Orthopedic Surgery, Jameson Crane Sports Medicine Institute, The Ohio State University, Columbus, Ohio

MOHAMED MARZOUK EL ARABY, MD
Department of Biomedical Sciences, Humanitas University, Humanitas Clinical and Research Center, Rozzano, Milan, Italy

LAWRENCE ENWEZE, MD
Department of Orthopedic Surgery, Stanford University, Redwood City, California

RACHEL M. FRANK, MD
Assistant Professor, Sports Medicine and Shoulder Surgery, Assistant Professor, Department of Orthopaedic Surgery, University of Colorado School of Medicine, Aurora, Colorado

ALAN GETGOOD, MPhil, MD, FRCS (Tr&Orth)
Consultant Orthopaedic Surgeon, Division of Orthopaedic Surgery, Western University, Fowler Kennedy Sports Medicine Clinic, 3M Centre, London, Ontario, Canada

ANDREAS H. GOMOLL, MD
Associate Professor of Orthopedic Surgery, Hospital for Special Surgery, Weill Cornell Medical School, New York, New York

KYLA HUEBNER, MSc, MD, PhD
Orthopaedic Resident, Division of Orthopaedic Surgery, Western University, Fowler Kennedy Sports Medicine Clinic, 3M Centre, London, Ontario, Canada

FRANCESCO IACONO, MD
Department of Biomedical Sciences, Humanitas University, Humanitas Clinical and Research Center, Rozzano, Milan, Italy

MITCHELL I. KENNEDY, BS
Clinical Outcomes-Based Orthopaedic Researcher, Steadman Philippon Research Institute, Vail, Colorado

ELIZAVETA KON, MD
Professor, Department of Biomedical Sciences, Humanitas University, Humanitas Clinical and Research Center, Rozzano, Milan, Italy

ROBERT F. LaPRADE, MD, PhD
Chief Medical Officer, Steadman Philippon Research Institute, Co-Director, Sports Medicine Fellowship Program, Physician, The Steadman Clinic, Vail, Colorado

ADRIAN D.K. LE, MD
Department of Orthopedic Surgery, Stanford University, Redwood City, California, USA; Medical Director, Lifemark Health, Toronto, Canada

MAURILIO MARCACCI, MD
Professor, Department of Biomedical Sciences, Humanitas University, Humanitas Clinical and Research Center, Rozzano, Milan, Italy

COLIN P. MURPHY, BA
Center for Orthopaedic Outcomes Research, Steadman Philippon Research Institute, Vail, Colorado

ALESSANDRA NANNINI, MD
Department of Biomedical Sciences, Humanitas University, Humanitas Clinical and Research Center, Rozzano, Milan, Italy

NEAL B. NAVEEN, BS
Department of Orthopedics, Rush University Medical Center, Chicago, Illinois

BENEDICT U. NWACHUKWU, MD, MBA
Department of Orthopedics, Rush University Medical Center, Chicago, Illinois

LIAM A. PEEBLES, BA
Center for Orthopaedic Outcomes Research, Steadman Philippon Research Institute, Vail, Colorado

MATTHEW T. PROVENCHER, MD
Captain, Medical Corps, US Naval Reserves, Center for Orthopaedic Outcomes Research, Steadman Philippon Research Institute, The Steadman Clinic, Vail, Colorado

STEFANO RESPIZZI, MD
Department of Biomedical Sciences, Humanitas University, Humanitas Clinical and Research Center, Rozzano, Milan, Italy

SCOTT A. RODEO, MD
Attending Orthopaedic Surgeon, Department of Sports Medicine and Shoulder, Hospital for Special Surgery, New York, New York

ANTHONY SANCHEZ, BS
Center for Orthopaedic Outcomes Research, Steadman Philippon Research Institute, Vail, Colorado, USA; School of Medicine, Oregon Health & Science University, Portland, Oregon

TAYLOR M. SOUTHWORTH, BS
Department of Orthopedics, Rush University Medical Center, Chicago, Illinois

NICOLÒ DANILO VITALE, MD
Department of Biomedical Sciences, Humanitas University, Humanitas Clinical and Research Center, Rozzano, Milan, Italy

KATHLEEN WEBER, MD, MS
Director of Primary Care and Sports Medicine, Assistant Professor, Department of Orthopaedics, Rush University Medical Center, Midwest Orthopaedics at Rush, Chicago, Illinois

NINA A. YAFTALI, DO
Fellow, Primary Care Sports Medicine, Rush University Medical Center, Midwest Orthopaedics at Rush, Chicago, Illinois

Contents

> Osteoarthritis is a common condition that affects many individuals resulting in pain, reduced mobility, and decreased function. Corticosteroids have been a mainstay of osteoarthritis treatment. Studies have shown that they provide short-term pain improvement and can be used for osteoarthritis flares. Hyaluronic acid injections have extensively been studied in knee osteoarthritis but to a lesser degree in other joints. Despite some debate between societies, a large number of recent studies have shown hyaluronic acid to be a viable treatment option showing longer-term improvement in both pain and function.

> Platelet-rich plasma (PRP) is a promising treatment for musculoskeletal maladies and clinical data to date have shown that PRP is safe. However, evidence of its efficacy has been mixed and highly variable depending on the specific indication. Additional future high-quality large clinical trials will be critical in shaping our perspective of this treatment option. The heterogeneity of PRP preparations, both presently and historically, leads sweeping recommendations about its utility impossible to make. This heterogeneity has also made interpreting existing literature more complicated.

> In orthopedic sports medicine, amniotic-derived products have demonstrated promising preclinical and early clinical results for the treatment of tendon/ligament injuries, cartilage defects, and osteoarthritis. The amniotic membrane is a metabolically active tissue that has demonstrated anti-inflammatory, antimicrobial, antifibrotic, and epithelialization-promoting features that make it uniquely suited for several clinical applications. Although the existing clinical literature is limited, there are several ongoing clinical trials aiming to elucidate the specific applications and benefits of these products. This article reviews the current amniotic-derived treatment options and the existing literature on outcomes, complications, and safety profile of these products for use in sports medicine.

> This article analyzes the current literature on the use of adipose-derived stem cells (ASCs) to evaluate the available evidence regarding their therapeutic potential in the treatment of cartilage pathology. Seventeen articles were included and analyzed, showing that there is overall a lack of high-quality evidence concerning the use of ASCs. Most trials are case series with short-term evaluation. The most adopted approach consists of an intra-articular injection of the stromal vascular fraction (SVF) rather than the expanded cells. Based on the available data, no specific preparation method or formulation could be considered as the preferred choice in clinical practice.

> Orthobiologics are a group of biological materials and substrates that promote bone, ligament, muscle, and tendon healing. These substances include bone autograft, bone allograft, demineralized bone matrix, bone graft substitutes, bone marrow aspirate concentrate, platelet-rich plasma, bone morphogenetic proteins, platelet-derived growth factor, parathyroid hormone, and vitamin D and calcium. Properties of orthobiologics in bone healing include osteoconduction, osteoinduction, and osteogenesis. This article discusses the important properties of orthobiologics in bone healing, many of the orthobiologics currently available for bone healing, the related literature, their current clinical uses in sports medicine, and systemic factors that inhibit bone healing.

> Biologics enhance tissue healing by stimulating the recovery processes for restoration of native or near-native tissue in addition to symptom management. The most popular biological modalities currently used include hyaluronic acid, growth factors therapy, platelet-rich plasma, and bone marrow aspirate concentrate. These treatment protocols are thought to facilitate and signal with cells or bioactive factors to improve ligament interventions by enhanced graft incorporation and strength, gene activation, and other mechanisms. Various growth factors regulate and improve cellular activities and proliferation, extracellular matrix deposition, and differentiation of mesenchymal stem cells into fibroblasts in the repair process of torn ligaments.

> Focal chondral defects of the knee are extremely common and often result in pain, dysfunction, joint deterioration, and, ultimately, the development of osteoarthritis. Due to the limitations of conventional treatments for focal

chondral defects of the knee, orthobiologics have recently become an area of interest. Orthobiologics used for cartilage defects include (but are not limited to) bone marrow aspirate concentrate, adipose-derived mesenchymal stem cells, platelet-rich plasma, and micronized allogeneic cartilage. Each of these products can be applied in the clinical setting, as an isolated surgical procedure, or as an augment to cartilage restoration surgery.

Osteoarthritis (OA) is a debilitation condition that affects millions of North Americans. Aside from weight loss, activity modification, and joint replacement, little else has been effective in delaying the progression of OA or treating the symptoms of OA. Ortho-biologics have become a popular treatment option in a variety of musculoskeletal conditions, including OA. In this article, the authors explore the use of 4 key ortho-biologics in the treatment of OA, all of which have shown promising results in the literature, despite the lack of large randomized controlled trials.

The future of orthopedic surgery appears to be intimately associated with the development of orthobiologics to facilitate healing and the treatment of multiple disease processes. The orthopedic community should understand developmental processes to ensure that products are adequately studied and the effects are fully known before widespread implementation in the clinical setting. Technologies that embrace this paradigm will impact the field the most.

The decision to incorporate ortho-biologics into a clinical practice will ultimately depend on physicians' preferences and the resources available to their practice. It is important to emphasize that different biologics are used for different pathologies/injuries and in different settings, such as the operating room or in the office. Physicians thinking about using biologics in their practices should consider the time commitment required to learn and use the technique, insurance coverage, and informed consent. The decision to treat patients with ortho-biologics should be a shared decision based on current literature, previous treatment regimen, and patients' goals.

OrthoBiologics in Sports Medicine

CLINICS IN SPORTS MEDICINE

SERIES OF RELATED INTERESTED

Orthopedic Clinics
Foot and Ankle Clinics
Hand Clinics
Physical Medicine and Rehabilitation Clinics
Clinics in Podiatric Medicine and Surgery

THE CLINICS ARE AVAILABLE ONLINE!
Access your subscription at:
www.theclinics.com

Foreword

OrthoBiologics: Science or Snake Oil?

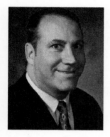

Mark D. Miller, MD
Consulting Editor

In many ways, the commercial appeal and financial benefits of OrthoBiologics, from joint juice to stem cells, has outpaced the science. Just browse the Internet or thumb through an airplane magazine and you can get a feel for the sensationalism that many institutes, providers, and industry have created about this topic. It is often difficult to sort out the science here. One problem is the tremendous placebo effect of many OrthoBiologic treatment options. Who would pay thousands of dollars for a treatment and then tell their friends (or admit to themselves) that it didn't work? Another problem is how to measure the effect of these treatments.

One key issue to sort out is what is rightly termed a "stem cell." Pluripotent cells can be obtained from blood, bone marrow, and even adipose tissue (who wouldn't be willing to give up some fat) and concentrated to yield higher numbers of these cells, but true stem cells need to be isolated and cultured to create meaningful numbers of true stem cells. And this cannot be done in the United States. To their credit, the Food and Drug Administration is policing this process, and we have all seen headlines about clinics that have been shut down for "manipulating" stem cells. Other countries do not have these restrictions, and some argue that this puts us at a disadvantage in treating our patients. We should all follow the results of OrthoBiologics in these less restricted countries and then advocate for policy change if efficacy and safety are proven.

In the interim, I recommend that we all put science first. This issue of *Clinics in Sports Medicine* is a great start. Drs Frank and Cole are international experts in this area and have invited an all-star group of authors to cover this important topic. I encourage you to read and understand each article and then keep up on the literature on this important topic. And...perhaps most importantly, consider the patient. It's not about how much

Clin Sports Med 38 (2019) xi–xii
https://doi.org/10.1016/j.csm.2018.09.004
0278-5919/19/© 2018 Published by Elsevier Inc.

sportsmed.theclinics.com

you can charge them (in almost all cases out of their own pockets), but how you can offer the best, scientifically proven, and reasonably priced treatment options to those individuals who have entrusted themselves to our care.

Thank you,

Mark D. Miller, MD
Division of Sports Medicine
Department of Orthopaedic Surgery
University of Virginia
James Madison University
400 Ray C. Hunt Drive, Suite 330
Charlottesville, VA 22908-0159, USA

E-mail address:
mdm3p@virginia.edu

Preface

OrthoBiologics in Sports Medicine: Real-Time Applications Are Here, and Future Developments Are Promising!

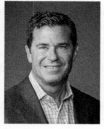 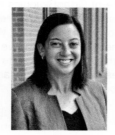

Brian J. Cole, MD, MBA   Rachel M. Frank, MD
Editors

OrthoBiologics have become increasingly utilized not only throughout the field of medicine but particularly in orthopedic surgery and sports medicine. The volume of literature describing products and techniques with a biologic basis has increased exponentially over the last several decades, with a variety of novel developments on the horizon. In this issue of *Clinics in Sports Medicine* we aim to bring our readers the most up-to-date information on OrthoBiologic techniques within sports medicine, utilizing a peer-reviewed format to ensure the information is accurate and reliable. While we hope that all literature can be thought of as accurate and reliable, this is of utmost importance when discussing novel biologic treatments, as the level of public misinformation is not insignificant. While many emerging therapies and techniques hold promise for improving function and reducing pain, a current product that has been proven to reproducibly regenerate damaged/diseased ligament, tendon, cartilage, and meniscus tissue, among other tissues, in a human population, unfortunately does not yet exist. Nevertheless, the field of OrthoBiologics is incredibly exciting, and the potential for tissue regeneration exists. In this issue of *Clinics in Sports Medicine*, multiple world-renowned experts summarize all available OrthoBiologic agents that have a role in the sports medicine patient population.

As many of the OrthoBiologic treatments that are described are administered via a local injection, Dr Kathy Weber begins this issue with a discussion of the most commonly utilized injection-based treatments for peri-articular and intra-articular conditions, including corticosteroid injections and viscosupplementation. Dr Jason Dragoo and colleagues then provide a comprehensive overview of platelet-rich

Clin Sports Med 38 (2019) xiii–xiv
https://doi.org/10.1016/j.csm.2018.09.003
0278-5919/19/© 2018 Published by Elsevier Inc.   **sportsmed.theclinics.com**

plasma. From here, a more focused discussion of more novel OrthoBiologic treatments ensues, with Dr Andreas Gomoll and coauthors discussing the amniotic-derived treatments and their typical utilization; Dr Elizaveta Kon and coauthors then summarizing adipose-derived stem cells; Dr Scott Rodeo and coauthors next discussing OrthoBiologics for bone healing; Dr Jorge Chahla and colleagues discussing OrthoBiologics for ligament repair and reconstruction; and Drs Rachel Frank and Brian Cole (your guest editors) and coauthors summarizing OrthoBiologics for focal chondral defects. Next, Dr Alan Getgood and colleagues describe the application of OrthoBiologics for the treatment of osteoarthritis, which, given the prevalence of osteoarthritis and its associated morbidity, will perhaps be one of the most clinically meaningful areas of OrthoBiologic application. Then, Dr Adam Anz and coauthors present emerging techniques and the future of OrthoBiologics in sports medicine, and finally, Dr Matthew Provencher and colleagues provide some real-life information on how to incorporate OrthoBiologics into your clinical practice. We hope that this collection of articles from this group of esteemed authors will prove useful for better understanding the real-time applications of OrthoBiologics in sports medicine, as well as the promising future developments being researched in basic, animal, translational, and clinical research studies around the globe.

Brian J. Cole, MD, MBA
Department of Orthopedics
Department of Surgery, Rush OPH
Midwest Orthopaedics at Rush
Sports Medicine and Surgery
Shoulder, Elbow and Knee Care
Cartilage Restoration Center at Rush
Rush University Medical Center
1611 West Harrison, Suite 300
Chicago, IL 60612, USA

Rachel M. Frank, MD
Sports Medicine and Shoulder Surgery
Department of Orthopaedic Surgery
University of Colorado School of Medicine
12631 East 17th Avenue
Mail Stop B202
Aurora, CO 80045, USA

E-mail addresses:
bcole@rushortho.com (B.J. Cole)
rachel.frank@ucdenver.edu (R.M. Frank)

Websites:
https://www.RachelFrankMD.com
http://www.BrianColeMD.com

Corticosteroids and Hyaluronic Acid Injections

Nina A. Yaftali, DO[a], Kathleen Weber, MD, MS[b],*

KEYWORDS

- Corticosteroid • Hyaluronic acid • Injections • Osteoarthritis • Efficacy
- Joint injection • Viscosupplementation

KEY POINTS

- Corticosteroid joint injections are commonly used in the treatment of pain associated with osteoarthritis.
- Studies have shown that corticosteroid injections provide short-term improvement in pain.
- Hyaluronic acid injections have been extensively studied in knee osteoarthritis and have shown efficacy in pain control and improved function, with many societies including hyaluronic acid injections as a part of their osteoarthritis treatment recommendations.
- The use of image guidance can improve accuracy of intraarticular placement of corticosteroids or hyaluronic acid injections.

Osteoarthritis (OA) is the most common form of arthritis and a frequent cause of disability in middle-aged and older adults leading to pain, reduced mobility, and loss of functionality.[1,2] It is estimated that 35% of patients older than 50 years[3] and up to 80% older than 65 years have OA.[3,4] Common nonpharmacologic treatment of OA includes weight loss, strengthening with or without formal physical therapy, activity modification, modalities, and some forms of bracing.[5,6] However, when nonpharmacologic approaches do not provide adequate symptom control, a variety of oral, topical, and intraarticular medications, as well as biological treatments, can be used in conjunction with the nonpharmacologic treatments (**Fig. 1**). The optimal conservative management of OA requires a combination of pharmacologic and nonpharmacologic treatment modalities to reduce pain, improve function, and potentially aid in limiting disease progression.[6] This article focuses on intraarticular corticosteroid and hyaluronic acid (HA) injections for the treatment of OA.

Dr Weber has received fund from Flexim Therapeutics.
^a Primary Care Sports Medicine, Rush University Medical Center, Midwest Orthopaedics at Rush, 1611 West Harrison, 3rd Floor, Chicago, IL 60612, USA; ^b Department of Orthopaedics, Rush University Medical Center, Midwest Orthopaedics at Rush, 1611 West Harrison, 3rd Floor, Chicago, IL 60612, USA
* Corresponding author.
E-mail address: kweber@rushortho.com

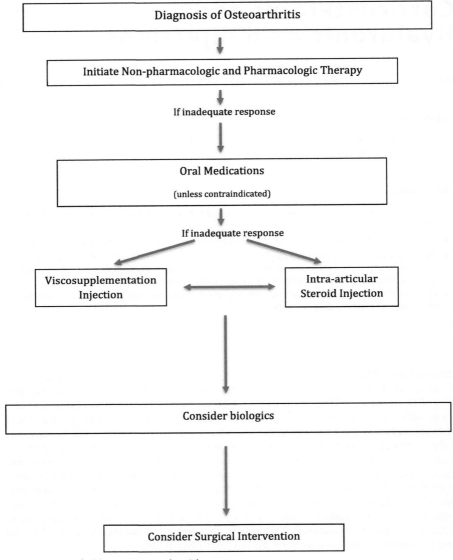

Fig. 1. Osteoarthritis treatment algorithm.

CORTICOSTEROIDS

Intraarticular corticosteroid injections (CSIs) were first established as treatment in OA and other rheumatologic conditions in 1951[7] and have been the mainstay of treatment over the decades. Understanding corticosteroids' mechanism of and duration of action, the different formulations, and the potential side effects is crucial when determining if the administration of a CSI is appropriate in the treatment of an individual's OA. CSIs are commonly used modalities in the treatment of symptomatic OA and produce both an antiinflammatory and an immunosuppressive effect.[6]

Mechanism of Action

The mechanism of action of corticosteroids is complex and has definitive local and possible systemic effects. Intraarticular CSIs act directly on nuclear steroid receptors, interrupting the inflammatory cascade. They interfere with the action of cytokines at different levels such as interleukin 1 (IL-1), tumor necrosis factor, IL-6, and IL-17, all of which are involved in the process of cartilage damage in OA.[8]

These injections work to reduce vascular permeability, inhibit secretion of inflammatory mediators such as prostaglandin and leukotriene, inhibit production of neutrophil superoxide as well as metalloproteinase, and downregulate immune function.[2,6,7,9]

Experimental animal models of OA suggest corticosteroids may reduce severity of cartilage lesions and size of osteophytes.[10,11] Clinically, the benefits from injections are known to provide pain relief and reduce joint effusions. Studies have shown that there are systemic benefits to intraarticular corticosteroids but these have mostly been studied in patients with rheumatoid arthritis with improvement in inflammatory markers, C-reactive protein, and erythrocyte sedimentation rate.[12,13]

Corticosteroid Preparations

There are currently multiple Food and Drug Administration (FDA)-approved corticosteroids for intraarticular injections. The preparations of steroids used in intraarticular injections are divided into 2 groups—particulate and nonparticulate (**Table 1**). Particulate steroids (nonwater soluble) such as methylprednisolone, betamethasone, and triamcinolone have a depot effect, resulting in a longer duration of action due to their ability to remain in the synovial fluid and the maintenance of continuous release of the active drug for longer periods of time.[12,14] The most commonly and widely used corticosteroid is methylprednisolone acetate, which has an average duration of action of 7 days.[7] In contrast, nonparticulate corticosteroids are water-soluble, smaller in particle size, and their crystals do not aggregate within the joint, leading to a shorter duration of action and rapid clearance from the joint.[14,15]

One of the newer available corticosteroids is triamcinolone acetonide extended release (ER), which was approved by the FDA in October 2017.[16] Triamcinolone acetonide ER uses microsphere technology to extend the analgesic effects of steroids at a therapeutic dose for several months.[17] One single intraarticular steroid injection has been found to produce significantly greater changes in daily pain score compared with placebo from weeks 1 to 12.[17] Further, the Western Ontario McMaster Universities Osteoarthritis Index (WOMAC) pain and functional limitation score was reduced compared with placebo.[17] Importantly, the phase II and III trials did not report any

Table 1
Formulations of corticosteroids

Particulate (Nonsoluble)	Nonparticulate (Soluble)
Betamethasone acetate	Betamethasone sodium phosphate
Hydrocortisone acetate	Dexamethasone acetate
Methylprednisolone acetate	
Prednisone tebutate	
Triamcinolone acetonide	
Triamcinolone acetonide ER	
Triamcinolone hexacetonide	

serious adverse effects and thus the potential benefits of this newer CSI are encouraging.[17]

Duration of Action

The duration of pain relief provided by the corticosteroid is unclear. The onset of action is quick—typically within 24 hours—whereas clinical relief can range from 2 weeks to up to 24 weeks in some individuals.[18] The Cochrane Database of Systematic Reviews[19] studied the effect of CSIs on knee OA. It showed that people who received intraarticular CSIs responded to treatment with a difference of 1.0 pain score in the visual analogue scale (VAS). Their impact in pain reduction was moderate at 1 to 2 weeks, small to moderate for weeks 4 to 6, and small at 13 weeks. The meta-analysis illustrated that intraarticular CSIs were more effective in function control, with a difference of functional score of 0.7 units. Effects were moderate at 4 to 6 weeks and negligible by 26 weeks. There was no difference with corticosteroid use regarding quality of life. In a double-blind randomized study by Gaffney and colleagues,[20] patients were treated with triamcinolone or placebo for knee OA. The patients who received CSI showed a statistically significant improvement in both VAS and functionality at their primary endpoints of 1 and 6 weeks. Meta-analysis by Godwin and Dawes[21] showed a clinically significant lower VAS score at 1 week, and pain reduction (no continuation of pain), and a significant pain reduction at 3 to 4 weeks. At 6 to 8 weeks, however, there was no difference in pain reduction or VAS score. A double-blind randomized study by Chao and colleagues[22] demonstrated significant decrease in pain and reduction of functionality at 4 and 12 weeks for patients without evidence of synovitis on ultrasound. Other studies support the use of CSIs reporting that they are effective in the short-term pain control and for acute osteoarthritic flares.[4,6,9,12,23–25]

Other factors that may influence the response of corticosteroids include the presence of a knee effusion and less radiographic evidence of OA. Both of these findings were noted to be a positive predictor of response to CSI potentially up to 24 weeks.[6,26] Conversely, factors such as obesity, chronic medical problems, and a sedentary lifestyle are negative predictors for a positive response to corticosteroids.[9]

Some studies have shown that various corticosteroids alone and in conjunction with local anesthetics led to cell death and have cytotoxic effects on the different cell types in vitro and in vivo.[27–29] A recent study by McAlindon and colleagues[30] reported that among patients with symptomatic knee OA, 2 years of intraarticular triamcinolone given every 3 months led to increased cartilage volume loss with no change in pain compared with saline. The loss of cartilage did not correlate with pain and symptom outcomes. In this study, patients' eligibility criteria included weight-bearing posterior-anterior and semiflexed radiographic Kellgren-Lawrence grade II or III OA and evidence of synovitis or an effusion on ultrasound. This large-scale study contrasted with other, smaller-scale medical publications. A study by Raynauld and colleagues,[10] for example, reported the opposite. In their double-blind trial, patients with Kellgren-Lawrence grade II to III OA without effusion were randomized to receive triamcinolone or saline every 3 months for 2 years. The investigators showed that there was no statistically significant difference between the mean joint space at 1 and 2 years, but there was a significant improvement in range of motion and night pain.[10] A comparison of both studies suggests that the presence of synovitis or intraarticular fluid may have contributed to accelerate cartilage loss.[30,31]

CSIs are commonly combined with an anesthetic such as lidocaine and bupivacaine. These anesthetics work by inhibiting nerve excitation through sodium-specific ion channels on neuronal cell membranes, thus causing local analgesia.[7]

The most common administered local anesthetic in musculoskeletal procedures is bupivacaine, due to its longer half-life and greater potency.[32] However, in certain in vitro studies, bupivacaine has shown to lead to more cell apoptosis compared with lidocaine.[3,33] This has altered some providers' use of bupivacaine in practice. These medications should be avoided in individuals with a known drug allergy to local anesthetics.

Intraarticular CSIs combined with local anesthetics are commonly administered for both diagnostic and therapeutic treatment of OA. The desired and expected effect immediately following the injection is immediate pain relief. If immediate or incomplete pain relief is not obtained, then either the injection was not placed intraarticularly or the source of pain is only in part intraarticular or not intraarticular at all. The use of fluoroscopy or ultrasound may improve accuracy of the injection placement.[34,35] If the injection does not provide the expected response, consideration of alternative differentials should be investigated.

Contraindications

CSIs can be beneficial but should be limited to patients without any known contraindications or prior adverse effects to these medications. One of the main contraindications to intraarticular steroid injection use is the presence of infection, including any potential overlying skin cellulitis, septic arthritis/bursitis, osteomyelitis, febrile illness, or systemic bacteremia.[36] Other contraindications are an unstable joint, intraarticular fracture, juxtaarticular osteoporosis, and uncontrolled bleeding disorders.[36] Corticosteroids are thought to inhibit bone healing, so they should be used with caution in the case of intraarticular fractures.[7] Caution should also be used with patients who are diabetic, on anticoagulants, immunosuppressed, or have a hemarthrosis.[36] Joint injection in the setting of coagulopathy or anticoagulant is controversial. Anticoagulation does not always need to be withheld before an intraarticular injection and should be determined on an individual's risk of bleeding and on a patient-to-patient basis. One study investigated patients who received injections for the shoulder and the knee while taking Coumadin, concluding that a mean international normalized ratio (INR) of 2.77 to 5 was safely tolerated,[37] whereas other investigators suggest holding anticoagulation in INR is greater than 2.[7] It may be helpful to work with prescribing physician to determine if anticoagulation needs to be held before receiving an intraarticular injection.

Side Effects

CSIs can manifest both systemic and local side effects. Most common are local side effects, including postinjection flare, infection, and local fat atrophy and/or skin hypopigmentation.[12,38,39] Injection flare is the most common side effect that can develop hours after injection and last up to 72 hours.[7] If the local inflammation increase lasts for more than 24 hours, a joint aspiration is recommended to exclude infection.[37] With appropriate sterile technique, the incidence of infection is as low as 0.01% to 0.03%, with some articles citing occurrence rates of 1 in 3000 up to 1 in 50,000.[40] Local tissue or fat atrophy typically occurs 1 to 4 months after an injection and is associated with inaccurate placement, less soluble agents, and a superficial injection.[24] Avascular necrosis has been reported on rare occasions, with the hip being the joint most commonly affected. Avascular necrosis has been associated with oral steroid use, comorbid conditions, and more often is idiopathic.[24]

Less commonly seen serious side effects include hemarthrosis, sepsis, and low-grade chronic infection. A retrospective cohort analysis by Xu and colleagues[41] looked at the characteristics of patients that suffered knee infections, defined as septic arthritis or chronic low-grade infection. The risk factors found were recent CSIs, increased body mass, injections performed by a general practitioner, and rheumatoid arthritis.

Although particulate intraarticular steroid injections are maintained locally, they can lead to systemic effects such as increased glucose levels and hypothalamic–pituitary–adrenal axis suppression. For diabetics, an intraarticular joint injection can lead to a hyperglycemic effect from 2 to 5 days after injection. Diabetics should be counseled on the potential for an increase in blood sugar and adjust their medications accordingly in consult with their endocrinologist or primary care physician.[42] A study done by Lazarevic and colleagues[40] showed that a single intraarticular injection of methylprednisolone shows a 21% decrease in serum cortisol levels 24 hours after injection, with adrenocorticotropic hormone levels returning to normal 1 to 4 weeks after injection.[12,40] For patients with adrenal problems or hypertension, intraarticular CSIs should be considered on a case-by-case basis.[7] Facial flushing has been reported in up to 15% of patients,[12] occurring on average 18 hours after injections and resolving within 36 hours without intervention.[13]

Recommendations for CSI for knee OA vary by organization, with no consensual agreement among the groups. In 2005, the American Academy of Orthopedic Surgery (AAOS) published an inconclusive recommendation for the use of CSIs in the treatment of knee OA.[43] They cited that there was a lack of compelling evidence of the benefits of it use. A meta-analysis and systemic review of corticosteroids use in knee OA by a Cochrane review[19] concluded that its use had low-quality evidence for long-term effect. This conclusion was based on the lack of evidence in support of functional improvement such as walking, stiffness, and quality of life.[6,18] Conversely, the American College of Rheumatology (ACR) in 2012 recommended CSIs in patients with knee OA who had failed full-dose acetaminophen.[44] The Osteoarthritis Research Society International Guidelines recommend intraarticular corticosteroids as short-term analgesia but physicians should consider other treatments for long-term management of OA.[45] The lack of consensus amongst the organization may be due to the short-term clinical response of corticosteroids and variable rates of improvement in pain and function.[23]

Effectiveness of CSIs for the treatment of OA of joints other than the knee is debated. The ACR and the European League against Rheumatism endorse CSIs for the hip joint for moderate OA.[44] A systemic review[46] on intraarticular hip injections suggests the likelihood of short-term pain reduction. The effect was largely reported at 1 week, similar to knee studies. Furthermore, recommendations for the use of intraarticular steroids for glenohumeral OA are based on knee studies, making it difficult for organizations to support its use. The AAOS is unable to recommend for or against its use in glenohumeral arthritis, citing inconclusive evidence.[47] A meta-analysis for intraarticular CSIs for carpometacarpal OA showed no difference in VAS pain score compared with placebo.[48]

VISCOSUPPLEMENTATION/HYALURONIC ACID

HA is a glycosaminoglycan molecule and is one of the main components of normal synovial fluid and cartilage extracellular matrix. It provides lubrication, shock absorption, and viscoelastic properties.[49] In OA, there is an age-related decrease in cellularity and glycosaminoglycan content that contributes to the weakening of the cartilage matrix.[1] Elevated levels of free radicals, inflammatory cytokines, and cleavage enzymes are found in the aging cartilage matrix.[19] High levels of these proinflammatories lead to the molecular fragment of HA. With aging there is a 33% to 50% reduction in HA concentration.[50] Viscosupplementation is thought to have an antiinflammatory effect on the synovial articular cartilage while improving lubricant and decreasing joint effusion.[1] A recent study by Shah and colleagues[51] using T1rho MR imaging showed an injection with high-molecular-weight viscosupplementation increased the quality of type II proteoglycan in cartilage cells. These findings suggest that HA improves the articular cartilage biochemistry in OA.[50] HA is thought to have chondroprotective effects, but these effects have only been studied in vitro.[49,50]

Viscosupplementation Preparations

There are numerous FDA-approved types of viscosupplementation for use in the United States (**Tables 2** and **3**). Each formula differs by its molecular weight, half-life, concentration, molecular structure, frequency, cost, and injection volume.[52] They are produced via harvested rooster comb or bacteria fermentation.[50,52] HA can be either low molecular weight, linear HA, or higher-molecular-weight reticulated HA.

Higher-molecular-weight HA is thought to have higher clinical efficacy, but these findings remain controversial.[52] Their increased clinical efficacy is believed to be because of a longer half-life in the joint.[49] A meta-analysis by Altman and colleagues[53] demonstrated that high-molecular-weight (greater than 3000 kDa) HA and those derived by biological fermentation showed a superior efficacy and safety profile. A systematic review by Colen and colleagues[54] compared different molecular weighted viscosupplements with placebo, with the investigators reporting a statistically significant decrease in VAS pain score at baseline and at 3 month follow-up for both groups. They were unable to recommend one type of viscosupplementation over another. An earlier meta-analysis by Ricci[55] reported no statistically significant difference between an intraarticular injection of high versus low-molecular-weight HA for knee OA. Notably, single-injection viscosupplementation treatment has not been found to be inferior to treatments requiring series of HA injections (ie, >1 injection to complete the treatment in a short period of time)[56,57]; however, single injection formulation efficacy has not been as extensively studied.

Onset of symptom improvement in HA is slower compared with CSI, but the analgesic effect of HA can last for weeks or months. A recent meta-analysis by Cochrane

Table 2
Bacterial hyaluronic acid injections

Brand Name	Description	Molecular Weight (Millions of Daltons)	Weekly Injections
Orthovisc (DepuyMitek)	High molecular wt. Hyaluronan	1–2.9	3
Hymovis (Fidia Pharma)	High molecular wt. Hyaluronan	0.5–0.73	2
Genvisc 850 (Orthogen)	Sodium hyaluronate	0.85	5
Gelsyn-3 (Bioventus)	Sodium Hyaluronate	1.1	3
Durolane (Bioventus)	Sodium hyaluronate	1	1
Euflexxa (Ferring Pharma)	Sodium hyaluronate	2.4–3.6	3
Monovisc (DePuy Synthes)	High molecular wt Hyaluronan	1.0–2.9	1

Table 3
Avian hyaluronic acid injections

Brand Name	Description	Molecular Wt (Millions of Daltons)	Weekly Injections (Millions of Daltons)
Synvisc (Sanofi-Aventis)	Hylan G-F 20	5.0–6.0	3
Supartz (Bioventus)	Sodium hyaluronate	0.62–1.17	3–5
Hyalgan (Fidia Pharma)	Sodium hyaluronate	0.5–0.73	3–5
Synvisc One (Sanofi-Aventis)	Hylan G-F 20	6	1
Gel one (Zimmer)	Cross-linked hyaluronate	N/A	1
Visco-3 (zimmer)	Sodium hyaluronate	0.62–1.17	3

Database Review[50] of viscosupplementation showed a series of 3 to 5 injections was efficacious by 4 weeks, reaching its maximum effectiveness at 8 weeks and lasting up to 24 weeks. This treatment led to an average duration of 5 to 13 weeks in its effects on pain and function after completing a course of injections, with some relief even lasting up to 1 year. HA had large effects between 4 and 24 weeks for pain and function compared with preinjection values.[50]

A study by Wang and colleagues[3] showed that HA limits the progression of knee OA after 2 years by reducing tibial cartilage volume loss and less increase in cartilage defect seen on MR imaging. A meta-analysis by Waddell and Bricker[58] showed that viscosupplementation can postpone total knee replacement with the median time for patients with Kellgren-Lawrence Grade 4 knee OA to progress to knee arthroplasty of 1.8 years. Other retrospective case reviews of patients with Kellgren-Lawrence Grade 4 OA treated with HA injections have shown a delay in surgery by a median time of 2 year.[30]

In a collection of pooled randomized trials, HA has been compared with placebo, nonsteroidal antiinflammatory drugs (NSAIDs), and CSIs. Specifically, a study by Bellamy and colleagues[50] compared HA, CSI, and placebo for the treatment of knee OA, and their study revealed statistically significant differences in the HA group compared with placebo at 4 weeks, with HA superior to CSI between 5 and 13 weeks. The HA group had a reduction in VAS score and WOMAC functionality at different periods throughout the study duration compared with various agents.[50] HA had comparable effects with NSAIDS but with fewer side effects.[50] In a separate study, Adams[59] evaluated HA alone, HA with NSAIDs, and NSAIDs alone, and they found that at 12 weeks there was significant difference in all 3 study groups from baseline, but no significant difference between the treatment groups. At 26 weeks, both HA groups showed a significant difference in pain and joint function over the NSAIDs alone. Notably, the HA with NSAIDs group had significant improvement in rest and night pain compared with HA alone at 26 weeks. A meta-analysis of randomized controlled trials of adults with symptomatic, radiographic knee OA by Bannuru and colleagues[60] analyzed the impact of multiple medications, including acetaminophen, diclofenac, ibuprofen, naproxen, celecoxib; intraarticular corticosteroids; HA injections; and oral and intraarticular placebo treatments. Their conclusion was that the most efficacious treatment for pain was intraarticular HA injections. For function, intraarticular HA was statistically better than intraarticular corticosteroid and intraarticular placebo injections.

Adverse Effects

Viscosupplementation typically has few serious adverse effects. Retrospective cohort study by Petrella and colleagues[61] reported that avian-derived HA had higher rates of adverse effects compared with nonavian HA. Adverse effects include postinjection flare, superficial itching, and headache. Postinjection flare involves joint swelling, warmth, and pain that usually resolves without any treatment within 72 hours.[56] Rare, more serious side effects can occur and include severe inflammatory reactions, pseudogout and pseudosepsis.[62] Petrella and colleagues[61] reported that with repeated injections, there is more of a risk of an adverse reaction, including pseudo-septic reactions. Pseudoseptic reactions are diagnosed by joint aspiration and treated with NSAIDs and/or intraarticular steroid injection, once a true joint infection has been ruled out. Several case reports of acute calcium pyrophosphate crystal disease after the second injection of Synvisc (Sanofi-Aventis) HA have been described.[63] The patients showed an increase in leukocytes, with a high percentage of neutrophils and calcium pyrophosphate dihydrate crystals, which was treated with NSAIDS.[63] Practitioners should be cognizant of the potential adverse effects and educate their patients accordantly.

HA viscosupplementation is recommended for patients who cannot tolerate adverse effects of pharmacologic therapies or who no longer respond adequately to nonpharmacologic therapies.[49] Although NSAIDs are commonly used and have been recommended for use in moderate pain associated with OA by ACR guidelines for the treatment of OA, they have potential for significant complications, particularly those affecting the gastrointestinal, renal, and cardiac organ systems.[44] For patients with noninflammatory OA, or elderly patients with contraindications to NSAIDS or limited ambulation, viscosupplementation is a viable alternative.[10] For younger patients or those individuals that have comorbid conditions that prohibit arthroplasty or otherwise do not wish to have surgery, HA may provide benefits while reducing pain and improving function. Although the ideal candidate for HA treatment has yet to be defined, the selection of appropriate candidates for viscosupplementation is crucial to achieve desired outcomes. There is some limited literature that discusses which patients are likely to have the best response to HA with respect to level of OA, age, sex, severity of symptoms, and/or physical activity levels.[52] Viscosupplementation may produce an improved response in early stage OA in patients older than 65 years.[23] Further, viscosupplementation should be considered in patients with knee OA who present with pain related to OA, have failed or have insufficient responses to or unable to tolerate oral medications and other nonpharmacologic therapies, or have comorbid conditions that prohibit surgery.

Recommendations supporting the use of HA in knee OA are mixed. The AAOS came out with a strong recommendation against the use of HA for patients with symptomatic OA of the knee in 2013.[64] Their recommendation was based on 14 studies, 5 of which did not show any meaningful clinical difference after treatment with HA, which was defined by 30% change in baseline. Of the 14 citied studies, half showed 18% to 45% improvement from baseline score with viscosupplementation and were comparable with NSAIDS and tramadol.[43] This recommendation is disputed among other organizations including the ACR, American Medical Society for Sports Medicine (AMSSM), and the Arthroscopic Association of North America (AANA). The ACR conditionally recommends HA injections for patients who had an inadequate response to initial therapy or failed first-line therapy such as physical therapy and NSAIDS.[44] The AMSSM performed a large meta-analysis that showed that patients who received HA compared with placebo or corticosteroids exhibited a statistically significant response to treatment.[65] The AANA has strong arguments against the notion that HA is inappropriate due to a large number of current studies supporting its use and the low incidence of adverse safety.[43]

Viscosupplementation Use in Other Osteoarthritic Joints

Hip
The vast majority of viscosupplementation studies have been related to knee OA. The studies describing the use of HA in hip OA have shown conflicting results. The ACR has cited no evidence in support of HA use in hip OA.[44] However, a meta-analysis showed evidence that HA works best in mild to moderate hip OA, with improvement as high as 40% to 60% compared with baseline, with results persisting for more than 3 months.[66] A meta-analysis by Lieberan and colleagues[67] demonstrated a decrease in pain VAS score by 2 with intraarticular HA hip OA injections but cited insufficient evidence to determine the length of the response.

Ankle
There are limited studies regarding the efficacy of the use of HA in ankle OA. Viscosupplementation is thought to be safe for use in OA of the ankle.[68] A systematic review by Chang and colleagues[68] was inconclusive regarding its effectiveness compared with corticosteroids, placebo, or conservative measures. A systematic literature review by Papalia and colleagues[69] showed a reduction in pain for both placebo- and HA-treated patients, with few adverse events. Chang and colleagues'[68] study revealed that the higher number of total injections (3 vs 1) led to more pain improvement, but the volume of HA was inversely proportional to pain relief, likely due to the small size of the ankle joint. This was in agreement with another study by Wittenevea and colleagues[70] that showed that 3 injections of HA provided more pain relief than 1.

Shoulder
The AAOS Treatment Guidelines[71] for glenohumeral OA state that viscosupplementation is a possible treatment option. Other studies have shown positive responses to high-molecular-weight HA, including improvements in pain reduction and improvements in activities of daily living in the setting moderate to severe glenohumeral arthritis following treatment.[72,73] Randomized, double-blind, placebo-controlled multi-centered trials in the United States have studied the safety and effectiveness of 3 injections of HA in the glenohumeral joint. In these studies, viscosupplementation injections were considered safe with no adverse effects, suggesting they can be used as a form of maintenance therapy in patients without committal rotator cuff pathology.[48,73,74]

Other joints
Intraarticular HA joint injections have been used in other small joints, but the outcomes associated with these treatments are not well studied. One study investigated HA use in small joints such as the carpometacarpal, intraphalangeal, and/or trapeziometacarpal joint of the hand, with the investigators concluding that the use of HA showed no difference compared with placebo.[48]

Injection Techniques

Proper needle placement and injection technique have been shown to correlate with better clinical outcomes.[75] Knee studies suggest that accuracy of medication placement varies by portal approach. Jackson and colleagues'[76] study supported a lateral midpatellar injection approach being intraarticular 93% of the time, versus the antero-medial (75%) and anterolateral (71%) approaches. Using fluoroscopic imaging,

Hussein[77] evaluated the accuracy of the standard sitting anterolateral portal approach versus a full-flexion anterolateral approach. His study revealed that only 74% of the anterolateral injections were placed on first attempt, whereas full-flexion anterolateral portal attempts were inside the joint 97.1% on first attempt. A radiographic study showed that 72% of blind hip injections were intraarticular.[75] In general, injections can be administered blind or by using image guidance depending on the operator's comfort. Many studies regarding the knee, hip, and glenohumeral joint demonstrate that ultrasound-guided injections are more accurate than landmark-based injection.[47,75,76] Fluoroscopic guidance with contrast can be used to assure intraarticular placement of the medication.[34]

SUMMARY

OA remains a significant source of disability, pain, and morbidity for many individuals. A combination of both nonpharmacologic and pharmacologic treatments should be implemented to achieve maximum benefit. A comprehensive conservative management approach should be adjusted and modified to optimize pain control and improve function. Knee studies have found CSIs to provide short-term pain improvement, whereas HA injections provide similar but longer pain control and improved function. Despite these medications being extensively studied in knee OA, the recommendation for their use varies between societies.

REFERENCES

1. Loeser RF, Goldring SR, Scanzello CR, et al. OA: a disease of the joint as an organ. Arthritis Rheum 2012;64(6):1697–707.
2. Malemud CJ, Islam N, Haqqi TM. Pathophysiological mechanisms in OA lead to novel therapeutic strategies. Cells Tissues Organs 2003;174(1–2):34–48.
3. Wang Y, Hall S, Hanna F, et al. Effects of Hylan G-F 20 supplementation on cartilage preservation detected by magnetic resonance imaging in OA of the knee: a two-year single-blind clinical trial. BMC Musculoskelet Disord 2011;12(1):195.
4. Neustadt DH. Intra-articular injections for OA of the knee. Cleve Clin J Med 2006; 73(10):897–8, 901–4, 906–11.
5. Conaghan PG, Dickson J, Grant RL. Care and management of OA in adults: summary of NICE guidance. BMJ 2008;336(7642):502–3.
6. Ayhan E, Kesmezacar H, Akgun I. Intraarticular injections (corticosteroid, hyaluronic acid, platelet rich plasma) for the knee OA. World J Orthop 2014;5.
7. MacMahon PJ, Eustace SJ, Kavanagh EC. Injectable corticosteroid and local anesthetic preparations: a review for radiologists. Radiology 2009;252(3):647–61.
8. Malemud CJ. Cytokines as therapeutic targets for OA. BioDrugs 2004;18(1): 23–35.
9. Uthman I, Raynauld J-P, Haraoui B. Intra-articular therapy in OA. Postgrad Med J 2003;79(934):449–53.
10. Raynauld J-P, Buckland-Wright C, Ward R, et al. Safety and efficacy of long-term intraarticular steroid injections in OA of the knee: a randomized, double-blind, placebo-controlled trial. Arthritis Rheum 2003;48(2):370–7.
11. Pelletier JP, Martel-Pelletier J, Cloutier JM, et al. Proteoglycan-degrading acid metalloprotease activity in human osteoarthritic cartilage, and the effect of intra-articular steroid injections. Arthritis Rheum 1987;30(5):541–8.
12. Cole BJ, Schumacher RHJ. Injectable corticosteroids in modern practice. J Am Acad Orthop Surg 2005;13(1):37–46.

13. Habib GS. Systemic effects of intra-articular corticosteroids. Clin Rheumatol 2009;28(7):749–56.
14. Makkar JK, Singh PM, Jain D, et al. Particulate vs non-particulate steroids for transforaminal epidural steroid injections: systematic review and meta-analysis of the current literature. Pain Physician 2016;19(6):327–40.
15. Derby R, Lee SH, Date ES, et al. Size and aggregation of corticosteroids used for epidural injections. Pain Med 2008;9(2):227–34.
16. Kaufman MB. Pharmaceutical approval update. P T 2017;42(12):733–55.
17. Bodick N, Lufkin J, Willwerth C, et al. An intra-articular, extended-release formulation of triamcinolone acetonide prolongs and amplifies analgesic effect in patients with OA of the knee: a randomized clinical trial. J Bone Joint Surg Am 2015;97(11):877–88.
18. Bellamy N, Campbell J, Welch V, et al. Intraarticular corticosteroid for treatment of OA of the knee. Cochrane Database Syst Rev 2006;(2):CD005328.
19. Jüni P, Hari R, Rutjes AWS, et al. Intra-articular corticosteroid for knee OA. Cochrane Database Syst Rev 2015;(10):CD005328.
20. Gaffney K, Ledingham J, Perry JD. Intra-articular triamcinolone hexacetonide in knee OA: factors influencing the clinical response. Ann Rheum Dis 1995;54(5):379–81.
21. Godwin M, Dawes M. Intra-articular steroid injections for painful knees. Systematic review with meta-analysis. Can Fam Physician 2004;50:241–8.
22. Chao J, Wu C, Sun B, et al. Inflammatory characteristics on ultrasound predict poorer longterm response to intraarticular corticosteroid injections in knee OA. J Rheumatol 2010;37(3):650–5.
23. Cheng OT, Souzdalnitski D, Vrooman B, et al. Evidence-based knee injections for the management of arthritis. Pain Med 2012;13(6):740–53.
24. Pekarek B, Osher L, Buck S, et al. Intra-articular corticosteroid injections: a critical literature review with up-to-date findings. Foot (Edinb) 2011;21(2):66–70.
25. Legré-Boyer V. Viscosupplementation: Techniques, indications, results. Orthop Traumatol Surg Res 2015;101(1, Supplement):S101–8.
26. Weitoft T, Uddenfeldt P. Importance of synovial fluid aspiration when injecting intra-articular corticosteroids. Ann Rheum Dis 2000;59(3):233–5.
27. Farkas B, Kvell K, Czömpöly T, et al. Increased chondrocyte death after steroid and local anesthetic combination. Clin Orthop Relat Res 2010;468(11):3112–20.
28. Karpie JC, Chu CR. Lidocaine exhibits dose- and time-dependent cytotoxic effects on bovine articular chondrocytes in vitro. Am J Sports Med 2007;35(10):1621–7.
29. Nakazawa F, Matsuno H, Yudoh K, et al. Corticosteroid treatment induces chondrocyte apoptosis in an experimental arthritis model and in chondrocyte cultures. Clin Exp Rheumatol 2002;20(6):773–81.
30. McAlindon TE, LaValley MP, Harvey WF, et al. Effect of intra-articular triamcinolone vs saline on knee cartilage volume and pain in patients with knee OA: a randomized clinical trial. JAMA 2017;317(19):1967–75.
31. Eckstein F, Boudreau RM, Wang Z, et al. Trajectory of cartilage loss within 4 years of knee replacement – a nested case–control study from the OA initiative. Osteoarthritis Cartilage 2014;22(10):1542–9.
32. Braun HJ, Wilcox-Fogel N, Kim HJ, et al. The effect of local anesthetic and corticosteroid combinations on chondrocyte viability. Knee Surg Sports Traumatol Arthrosc 2012;20(9):1689–95.
33. Chu CR, Izzo NJ, Papas NE, et al. In vitro exposure to 0.5% bupivacaine is cytotoxic to bovine articular chondrocytes. Arthroscopy 2006;22(7):693–9.

34. Shortt CP, Morrison WB, Roberts CC, et al. Shoulder, hip, and knee arthrography needle placement using fluoroscopic guidance: practice patterns of musculoskeletal radiologists in North America. Skeletal Radiol 2009;38(4):377–85.

35. Schumacher HR. Aspiration and injection therapies for joints. Arthritis Care Res 2003;49(3):413–20.

36. J Monseau A, Singh Nizran P. Common injections in musculoskeletal medicine. Prim Care 2013;40(4):987–1000.

37. Bashir MA, Ray R, Sarda P, et al. Determination of a safe INR for joint injections in patients taking warfarin. Ann R Coll Surg Engl 2015;97(8):589–91.

38. Okere K, Jones MC. A case of skin hypopigmentation secondary to a corticosteroid injection. South Med J 2006;99(12):1393–4.

39. Loarte Pasquel EP, Cabal García AA. Cutaneous atrophy and hypopigmentation secondary to intra-articular corticosteroid injection. Semergen 2014;40(3):e61–3 [in Spanish].

40. Lazarevic MB, Skosey JL, Djordjevic-Denic G, et al. Reduction of cortisol levels after single intra-articular and intramuscular steroid injection. Am J Med 1995; 99(4):370–3.

41. Xu C, Peng H, Li R, et al. Risk factors and clinical characteristics of deep knee infection in patients with intra-articular injections: a matched retrospective cohort analysis. Semin Arthritis Rheum 2018;47(6):911–6.

42. Black DM, Filak AT. Hyperglycemia with non-insulin-dependent diabetes following intraarticular steroid injection. J Fam Pract 1989;28(4):462–3.

43. Brown GA. AAOS clinical practice guideline: treatment of OA of the knee: evidence-based guideline, 2nd Edition. J Am Acad Orthop Surg 2013;21(9): 577–9.

44. Hochberg MC. American College of Rheumatology 2012 recommendations for the use of nonpharmacologic and pharmacologic therapies in OA of the hand, hip, and knee. Arthritis Care Res (Hoboken) 2012;64(4):465–74.

45. Wehling P, Evans C, Wehling J, et al. Effectiveness of intra-articular therapies in OA: a literature review. Ther Adv Musculoskelet Dis 2017;9(8):183–96.

46. McCabe PS, Maricar N, Parkes MJ, et al. The efficacy of intra-articular steroids in hip OA: a systematic review. Osteoarthritis Cartilage 2016;24(9):1509–17.

47. Gross C, Dhawan A, Harwood D, et al. Glenohumeral joint injections: a review. Sports Health 2013;5(2):153–9.

48. Kroon FPB, Rubio R, Schoones JW, et al. Intra-articular therapies in the treatment of hand OA: a systematic literature review. Drugs Aging 2016;33(2):119–33.

49. Waddell DD. Viscosupplementation with hyaluronans for OA of the knee. Drugs Aging 2007;24(8):629–42.

50. Bellamy N, Campbell J, Robinson VA, et al. Viscosupplementation for the treatment of OA of the knee. Cochrane Database Syst Rev 2005;(2):CD005321.

51. Shah RP, Stambough JB, Fenty M, et al. T1rho magnetic resonance imaging at 3T detects knee cartilage changes after viscosupplementation. Orthopedics 2015; 38(7):e604–10.

52. Bowman S, Awad ME, Hamrick MW, et al. Recent advances in hyaluronic acid based therapy for OA. Clin Transl Med 2018;7(1):6.

53. Altman RD, Bedi A, Karlsson J, et al. Product differences in intra-articular hyaluronic acids for OA of the knee. Am J Sports Med 2016;44(8):2158–65.

54. Colen S, van den Bekerom MP, Mulier M, et al. Hyaluronic acid in the treatment of knee OA: a systematic review and meta-analysis with emphasis on the efficacy of different products. BioDrugs 2012;26(4):257–68.

55. Ricci M. Clinical comparison of oral administration and viscosupplementation of hyaluronic acid (HA) in early knee OA. Musculoskelet Surg 2017;101(1):45–9.

56. Newberry SJ, Fitzgerald JD, Maglione MA, et al. Systematic review for effectiveness of hyaluronic acid in the treatment of severe degenerative joint disease (DJD) of the knee. Rockville (MD): Agency for Healthcare Research and Quality (US); 2015.

57. Gigis I, Fotiadis E, Nenopoulos A, et al. Comparison of two different molecular weight intra-articular injections of hyaluronic acid for the treatment of knee OA. Hippokratia 2016;20(1):26–31.

58. Waddell DD, Bricker DC. Total knee replacement delayed with Hylan G-F 20 use in patients with grade IV OA. J Manag Care Pharm 2007;13(2):113–21.

59. Adams ME. The role of viscosupplementation with hylan G-F 20 (Synvisc) in the treatment of OA of the knee: a Canadian multicenter trial comparing hylan G-F 20 alone, hylan G-F 20 with non-steroidal anti-inflammatory drugs (NSAIDs) and NSAIDs alone. Osteoarthr Cartil 1995;3(4):213–25.

60. Bannuru RR, Schmid CH, Kent DM, et al. Comparative effectiveness of pharmacologic interventions for knee OA: a systematic review and network meta-analysis. Ann Intern Med 2015;162(1):46–54.

61. Petrella R, Cogliano A, Decaria J. Comparison of avian and nonavian hyaluronic acid in OA of the knee. Orthop Res Rev 2010;2:5–9.

62. Danilkowicz R, Robinson M, Steffes M, et al. Inflammatory pseudoseptic reaction to synvisc-one injection requiring diagnostic arthroscopy. J Case Rep Images Orthop Rheum 2017;2:7–11.

63. Kroesen S, Schmid W, Theiler R. Induction of an acute attack of calcium pyrophosphate dihydrate arthritis by intra-articular injection of hylan G-F 20 (Synvisc). Clin Rheumatol 2000;19(2):147–9.

64. Jevsevar DS. Treatment of OA of the knee: evidence-based guideline, 2nd Edition. J Am Acad Orthop Surg 2013;21(9):571–6.

65. Trojian TH, Concoff AL, Joy SM, et al. AMSSM scientific statement concerning viscosupplementation injections for knee OA: importance for individual patient outcomes. Br J Sports Med 2016;50(2):84–92.

66. Migliore A, Anichini S. Intra-articular therapy in hip OA. Clin Cases Miner Bone Metab 2017;14(2):179–81.

67. Lieberman JR, Engstrom SM, Solovyova O, et al. Is intra-articular hyaluronic acid effective in treating OA of the hip joint? J Arthroplasty 2015;30(3):507–11.

68. Chang K-V, Hsiao M-Y, Chen W-S, et al. Effectiveness of intra-articular hyaluronic acid for ankle OA treatment: a systematic review and meta-analysis. Arch Phys Med Rehabil 2013;94(5):951–60.

69. Papalia R, Albo E, Russo F, et al. The use of hyaluronic acid in the treatment of ankle OA: a review of the evidence. J Biol Regul Homeost Agents 2017;31(4 Suppl 2):91–102.

70. Witteveen AG, Giannini S, Guido G, et al. A prospective multi-centre, open study of the safety and efficacy of hylan G-F 20 (Synvisc) in patients with symptomatic ankle (talo-crural) OA. Foot Ankle Surg 2008;14(3):145–52.

71. Silverstein E, Leger R, Shea KP. The use of intra-articular hylan G-F 20 in the treatment of symptomatic OA of the shoulder: a preliminary study. Am J Sports Med 2007;35(6):979–85.

72. Di Giacomo G, de Gasperis N. Hyaluronic acid intra-articular injections in patients affected by moderate to severe glenohumeral OA: a prospective randomized study. Joints 2017;5(3):138–42.

73. Kwon YW, Eisenberg G, Zuckerman JD. Sodium hyaluronate for the treatment of chronic shoulder pain associated with glenohumeral OA: a multicenter, randomized, double-blind, placebo-controlled trial. J Shoulder Elbow Surg 2013;22(5): 584–94.
74. Blaine T, Moskowitz R, Udell J, et al. Treatment of persistent shoulder pain with sodium hyaluronate: a randomized, controlled trial. A multicenter study. J Bone Joint Surg Am 2008;90(5):970–9.
75. Hoeber S, Aly A-R, Ashworth N, et al. Ultrasound-guided hip joint injections are more accurate than landmark-guided injections: a systematic review and meta-analysis. Br J Sports Med 2016;50(7):392–6.
76. Jackson DW, Evans NA, Thomas BM. Accuracy of needle placement into the intra-articular space of the knee. J Bone Joint Surg Am 2002;84-A(9):1522–7.
77. Hussein M. An accurate full-flexion anterolateral portal for needle placement in the knee joint with dry OA. J Am Acad Orthop Surg 2017;25(7):e131–7.

Platelet-Rich Plasma

Adrian D.K. Le, MD, Lawrence Enweze, MD, Malcolm R. DeBaun, MD,
Jason L. Dragoo, MD*

KEYWORDS

- Platelet-rich plasma • PRP • Orthobiologics • Regenerative medicine
- Tendinopathy • Osteoarthritis • Augmentation

KEY POINTS

- There is abundant high-quality level I evidence to recommend leukocyte-rich platelet-rich plasma (LR-PRP) injections for lateral epicondylitis and LP-PRP injections for osteoarthritis of the knee.
- There is a moderate amount of high-quality level I evidence to recommend LR-PRP injections for patellar tendinopathy and PRP injections for plantar fasciitis.
- There is currently insufficient high-quality evidence for recommendation, but small clinical trials have shown promising efficacy for PRP injections for rotator cuff tendinopathy, osteoarthritis of the hip, donor site pain in anterior cruciate ligament (ACL) reconstruction with patellar tendon autograft, and LP-PRP injections for high ankle sprains.
- The best available clinical evidence does not demonstrate efficacy of PRP injections for Achilles tendinopathy, acute fracture, or nonunion; surgical augmentation with PRP in rotator cuff repair, Achilles tendon repair, and ACL reconstruction; and efficacy has not been shown with PRP injections for muscle injuries, although preclinical studies suggest platelet-poor plasma may hold promise for muscle injuries, but clinical trials will be necessary to validate this.

INTRODUCTION

Platelet-rich plasma (PRP) is an autologous concentration of human platelets in a small volume of plasma produced by centrifuging a patient's own blood. Platelets contain a milieu of growth factors and mediators in their alpha granules (transforming growth factor [TGF]-β1, platelet-derived growth factor, basic fibroblast growth factor, vascular endothelial growth factor, epidermal growth factor, insulinlike growth factor [IGF]-1),[1,2] which are concentrated through the centrifugation process and then be delivered to an injury site to augment the body's natural healing process.[3] The normal human platelet count ranges anywhere from 150,000 to 350,000/μL. Improvements in

Disclosure Statement: None (A.D.K. Le, L. Enweze, M.R. DeBaun). J.L. Dragoo – per the American Academy of Orthopaedic Surgeons Web site.
Department of Orthopedic Surgery, Stanford University, 450 Broadway Street, Redwood City, CA 94063, USA
* Corresponding author.
E-mail address: jdragoo@stanford.edu

bone and soft tissue healing properties have been demonstrated with concentrated platelets of 1,000,000/μL, and thus it is this concentration of platelets in a 5-mL volume of plasma that has been suggested as one working definition of PRP.[2,4] Another proposed definition of PRP is any plasma fraction that concentrates platelets greater than baseline. A resultant threefold to fivefold increase in growth and differentiation factors can be expected with PRP compared with normal nonconcentrated whole blood. PRP preparations are typically further categorized into leukocyte-rich PRP (LR-PRP) preparations, defined as having a neutrophil concentration above baseline, and leukocyte-poor PRP (LP-PRP) preparations, defined as having a leukocyte (neutrophil) concentration below baseline.

PREPARATION AND COMPOSITION

Currently more than 16 commercial PRP systems are available on the market, and hence quite a bit of variation exists in the PRP collection and preparation protocol depending on the commercial system being used (**Table 1**), which gives each system's PRP unique properties.[1,7–9] Each commercial system has a different platelet capture efficiency that results in different whole-blood volume requirements to achieve the necessary final platelet concentration for PRP. The commercial systems may also differ in their isolation method (1-step or 2-step centrifugation), the speed of centrifugation, and the type of collection tube system and operation. Generally, whole blood is usually collected and mixed with an anticoagulant factor, such as acid-citrate-dextrose, sodium citrate, or ethylene diamine tetra-acetic acid. Centrifugation then separates red blood cells (RBCs) from platelet-poor plasma (PPP) and the "buffy coat," which contains the concentrated platelets ± leukocytes. The platelet-concentrated layer is isolated using various processing techniques, and the RBC and PPP layers may be discarded. The platelets can then be directly injected into the patient or be "activated" via the addition of either calcium chloride or thrombin, which then causes the platelets to degranulate and release the growth and differentiation factors. Approximately 70% of the stored growth factors are released within the first 10 minutes of activation, and nearly 100% of the growth factors are released within 1 hour of activation.[2,4] Small amounts of growth factors may continue to be produced by the platelet during the remainder of its life span (8–10 days).

The specific composition of PRP, however, likely varies not only from person to person but also when the isolation process is repeated in the same individual.[9] Both patient-specific factors, including medications taken, and commercial system preparation methods are known to influence the specific makeup of PRP.[8–10] The variability in the cellular composition of PRP preparations creates challenges in interpretation of the literature regarding the clinical efficacy of PRP.

Our current understanding appears to suggest that PRP with elevated leukocyte content, that is, leukocyte (neutrophil)-rich PRP (LR-PRP), is associated with proinflammatory effects.[8] The elevated leukocyte (neutrophil) concentrations present in LR-PRP are also associated with elevated catabolic cytokines, such as interleukin (IL)-1β, tumor necrosis factor (TNF)-α, and metalloproteinases,[10,11] which may antagonize the anabolic cytokines contained within platelets. The clinical ramifications and cellular effects of these different PRP preparations, including leukocyte content, are still currently being elucidated. To better evaluate and summarize the best quality evidence available for various clinical indications for different PRP preparations, we have performed a systematic review of the literature, and present our methods and results in the following sections.

Table 1
Characteristics of PRP preparations from different commercially available systems

System	Company	Blood Volume Required, mL	Concentrated Volume Produced, mL	Processing Time, min	PPP Produced?	Increase in [Platelets], Times Baseline	Platelet Capture Efficiency, % Yield
Leukocyte-rich PRP							
Angel	Arthrex (Florida, USA)	52[5]	1–20[a]	17[5]	+	10[a]	56%–75%[5]
GenesisCS	EmCyte (Florida, USA)	54[5]	6[5]	10[5]	+	4–7[5]	61% ± 12%[5]
GPS III	Biomet (Now known as Zimmer Biomet, Indiana, USA)	54[5]	6[5]	15[5]	+	3–10[5]	70% ± 30%[5]
Magellan	Isto Biologics/Arteriocyte (Now known as Isto Biologics, Massachusetts, USA)	52[5]	3.5–7[5]	17[5]	+	3–15[5]	86% ± 41%[5]
SmartPReP 2	Harvest (Now known as Terumo BCT, Colorado, USA)	54[5]	7[5]	14[5]	+	5–9[5]	94% ± 12%[5]
Leukocyte-poor PRP							
Autologous Conditioned Plasma (ACP)	Arthrex	11[6]	4[6]	5[6]	–	1.3[6]	48% ± 7%[6]
Cascade	MTF (New Jersey, USA)	18[7]	7.5[7]	6[7]	–	1.6[7]	68% ± 4%[7]
Clear PRP	Harvest	54[a]	6.5[a]	18[a]	+	3–6[a]	62% ± 5%[a]
Pure PRP	EmCyte	50[a]	6.5[a]	8.5[a]	+	4–7[a]	76% ± 4%[a]

Abbreviations: PPP, platelet-poor plasma; PRP, platelet-rich plasma.
Plus minus sign signifies reported variance of platelet capture efficiency.
[a] Data obtained from manufacturers' promotional literature or internal studies.

TREATMENT OF TENDON INJURIES

PRP has been most actively evaluated in the treatment of tendon injuries or tendinopathies (**Table 2**). Tendons and ligaments heal through a dynamic process, with stages of inflammation, cellular proliferation, and subsequent tissue remodeling. Many of the cytokines found in PRP are involved in the signaling pathways that occur during this restorative process.[1,2] PRP may also promote neovascularization, which may not only increase the blood supply and nutrients needed for cells to regenerate the injured tissue, but may also bring new cells and remove debris from damaged tissue. Both these mechanisms of action are particularly attractive in chronic tendinopathy conditions in which the biologic milieu may be unfavorable for tissue healing. A recent systematic review and meta-analysis by Miller and colleagues[42] concluded that injections of PRP were more efficacious than control injections for treatment of symptomatic tendinopathy.

Lateral Epicondylitis

Clinical studies have evaluated PRP in lateral epicondylitis for patients who have failed to respond to physical therapy. In the largest such study, Mishra and colleagues[20] evaluated 230 patients who failed to respond to at least 3 months of conservative treatment for lateral epicondylitis in a prospective cohort study. Patients were treated with LR-PRP and at 24 weeks, the patients who received LR-PRP reported a 71.5% improvement in their pain scores compared with a 56.1% improvement in the control group (P = .019). The percentage of patients reporting significant residual elbow tenderness at 24 weeks was 29.1% in the patient group receiving PRP compared with 54.0% in the control group (P = .009). There was a clinically meaningful and statistically significant improvement at 24 weeks in patients treated with LR-PRP versus active control injection of local anesthetic.

PRP may also provide longer continuous relief of symptoms for lateral epicondylitis than corticosteroid injection and therefore have a more sustainable treatment effect. Gosens and colleagues[17] and Peerbooms and colleagues[43] evaluated the efficacy of LR-PRP versus corticosteroids in 100 patients who had a minimum 6-month history of recalcitrant chronic epicondylitis and had failed to respond to conservative management. Treatment success within this study was defined as, at minimum, a 25% reduction in the visual analog scale (VAS) score or Disability of Arm, Shoulder, and Hand score without a repeat intervention after 1 year. Although both groups improved in VAS scores from baseline, 73% (37 of 51 patients) in the PRP group versus 49% (24 of 49 patients) in the corticosteroid group were considered to have a successful response at 1 year (P<.001). Furthermore, 73% (37 of 51 patients) in the PRP group versus 51% (25 of 49 patients) in the corticosteroid group noted improved Disability of Arm, Shoulder, and Hand scores at 1 year (P = .005). Patients who received PRP also continued to report symptom relief 1 year after receiving the injection, whereas the short-term benefits of corticosteroids began to wane after 12 weeks. The improvement within this group of patients who received PRP continued to be noted 2 years after the PRP injection.[17]

- Summary and Recommendations: PRP is an effective treatment for lateral epicondylitis, with high-quality evidence demonstrating short-term and long-term efficacy. This recommendation also has been supported by previous reviews[42,44,45] and best available evidence specifically suggests LR-PRP should be the treatment of choice.

Patellar Tendinopathy

Results from randomized controlled trials (RCTs) appear to support the use of LR-PRP to treat chronic refractory patellar tendinopathy. Dragoo and colleagues[25] evaluated

Table 2
Study design characteristics for PRP versus control injection for tendinopathies

Indication	Study and Year of Publication	Level of Evidence	Sample Size PRP	Sample Size Control	Type of PRP	Number of Injections	Intervention/Injection Volume and Contents PRP	Intervention/Injection Volume and Contents Control	Follow-up, mo	Favors PRP?
Achilles tendinopathy	Boesen et al,[12] 2017	I	20	20	LP-PRP	4	4 mL PRP + eccentric training	Sham injection + eccentric training	6	+
Achilles Tendinopathy	de Jonge et al,[13] 2011	I	27	27	LR-PRP	1	4 mL PRP	4 mL normal saline	12	−
Achilles tendinopathy	Krogh et al,[14] 2016	I	12	12	LR-PRP	1	10–15 mL lidocaine → 6 mL PRP	10–15 mL lidocaine → 6 mL normal saline	3	−
Lateral epicondylitis	Behera et al,[15] 2015	I	15	10	LP-PRP	1	3 mL PRP + .5 mL calcium chloride	3 mL bupivacaine + 0.5 mL normal saline	12	+
Lateral epicondylitis	Gautam et al,[16] 2015	I	15	15	LP-PRP	1	2 mL PRP	2 mL methylprednisolone	6	+
Lateral epicondylitis	Gosens et al,[17] 2011	I	51	49	LR-PRP	1	3 mL PRP	3 mL triamcinolone	24	+
Lateral epicondylitis	Krogh et al,[18] 2013	I	20	20	LR-PRP	1	10–15 mL lidocaine → 3 mL PRP	10–15 mL lidocaine → 1 mL triamcinolone + 2 mL lidocaine	3	−
Lateral epicondylitis	Lebiedzinski et al,[19] 2015	I	64	56	LP-PRP	1	3 mL PRP	1 mL betamethasone + 2 mL lidocaine	12	+
Lateral epicondylitis	Mishra et al,[20] 2013	II	112	113	LR-PRP	1	Bupivacaine → 2–3 mL PRP	Bupivacaine → 2–3 mL bupivacaine	6	+
Lateral epicondylitis	Montalvan et al,[21] 2016	I	25	25	LP-PRP	2	2 mL lidocaine → 2 mL PRP	2 mL lidocaine → 2 mL normal saline	12	−
Lateral epicondylitis	Palacio et al,[22] 2016	I	20	20	LP-PRP	1	3 mL PRP	3 mL dexamethasone	6	−
Lateral epicondylitis	Stenhouse et al,[23] 2013	I	15	13	LP-PRP	2	1–2 mL lidocaine → 2 mL PRP	1–2 mL lidocaine	6	−

(continued on next page)

Table 2
(continued)

Indication	Study and Year of Publication	Level of Evidence	Sample Size PRP	Sample Size Control	Type of PRP	Number of Injections	Intervention/Injection Volume and Contents PRP	Intervention/Injection Volume and Contents Control	Follow-up, mo	Favors PRP?
Lateral epicondylitis	Yadav et al,[24] 2015	I	30	30	LR-PRP	1	1 mL PRP	1 mL methylprednisolone	3	+
Patellar tendinopathy	Dragoo et al,[25] 2014	I	10	13	LR-PRP	1	3 mL bupivacaine → 6 mL PRP + dry needling	3 mL bupivacaine + dry needling	6	+
Patellar tendinopathy	Vetrano et al,[26] 2013	I	23	23	NR	2	2 mL PRP	Extracorporeal shock wave therapy	12	+
Plantar fasciitis	Acosta-Olivo et al,[27] 2016	I	14	14	NR	1	3 mL of PRP + .45 mL of 10% calcium gluconate + lidocaine	2 mL dexamethasone + 2 mL of lidocaine	4	−
Plantar fasciitis	Aksahin et al,[28] 2012	II	30	30	LR-PRP	1	3 mL PRP + 2 mL prilocaine	2 mL methylprednisolone + 2 mL prilocaine	6	−
Plantar fasciitis	Jain et al,[29] 2015	I	30	30	LR-PRP	1	2.5 mL PRP	1 mL triamcinolone + levobupivacaine + sodium bicarbonate	12	−
Plantar fasciitis	Jain et al,[30] 2018	II	40	40	LR-PRP	1	2 mL lidocaine → 3 mL PRP	2 mL methylprednisolone + 2 mL lidocaine	6	−
Plantar fasciitis	Mahindra et al,[31] 2016	I	25	25	NR	1	2.5–3 mL PRP	2 mL methylprednisolone	3	+
Plantar fasciitis	Monto,[32] 2014	I	20	20	LR-PRP	1	3 mL PRP + 6 mL bupivacaine	1 mL methylprednisolone + 6 mL bupivacaine	24	+
Plantar fasciitis	Omar et al,[33] 2012	II	15	15	NR	1	NR PRP	NR corticosteroid	1	+
Plantar fasciitis	Say et al,[34] 2014	II	25	25	NR	1	2.5 mL of PRP + 5.5% calcium chloride	1 mL methylprednisolone + 1 mL of prilocaine	6	+

Condition	Study				PRP type		Intervention	Control	Follow-up	Favors PRP
Plantar fasciitis	Sherpy et al,[35] 2015	—	25	25	LR-PRP	1	PRP + mepivacaine	1 mL triamcinolone + mepivacaine	3	–
Plantar fasciitis	Shetty et al,[36] 2014	II	30	30	LR-PRP	1	8 mL PRP	1 mL triamcinolone + 3 mL lidocaine	3	+
Plantar fasciitis	Tiwari et al,[37] 2013	I	30	30	LR-PRP	1	5 mL PRP	1 mL methylprednisolone + 1 mL prilocaine	6	+
Plantar fasciitis	Vahdatpour et al,[38] 2016	I	16	16	LR-PRP	1	3 mL PRP	1 mL methylprednisolone + 1 mL lidocaine	6	+
Rotator cuff tendinopathy	Kesikburun et al,[39] 2013	I	20	20	LR-PRP	1	1 mL lidocaine → 5 mL PRP	1 mL lidocaine → 5 mL normal saline	12	–
Rotator cuff tendinopathy	Rha et al,[40] 2013	I	20	19	LR-PRP	2	<1 mL lidocaine → 3 mL PRP	<1 mL lidocaine	6	+
Rotator cuff tendinopathy	Shams et al,[41] 2016	I	20	20	LP-PRP	1	2–2.5 mL PRP	5 mL triamcinolone	6	–

Abbreviations: →, denotes sequential injection; LP-PRP, leukocyte-poor PRP; LR-PRP, leukocyte-rich PRP; NR, not reported; PRP, platelet-rich plasma. +, indicates that the trial found in favor of PRP; –, indicates the trial did not favor of PRP.

23 patients with patellar tendinopathy on examination and MRI who had failed conservative management. Patients were randomized to receive ultrasound-guided dry needling alone or with injection of LR-PRP. Patients were followed for more than 26 weeks. At 12 weeks, the PRP group had improved, as measured by Victorian Institute of Sports Assessment, Patellar Tendon (VISA-P) score, significantly more than the dry needling group (P = .02). However, the difference was not significant at more than 26 weeks (P = .66), suggesting that the benefit of PRP for patellar tendinopathy may be *earlier* improvement of symptoms. Vetrano and colleagues[26] also reported the benefit of PRP injections for treatment of chronic refractory patellar tendinopathy. Forty-six patients with ultrasound-confirmed chronic unilateral patellar tendinopathy were randomized to receive either 2 PRP injections over 2 weeks or 3 sessions of focused extracorporeal shock wave therapy (ECSWT). Although there was no significant difference between groups at 2-month follow-up, the PRP group showed statistically significant improvement, as measured by VISA-P and VAS, over ECSWT at 6-month and 12-month follow-up, and as measured by Blazina scale score at 12-month follow-up (P<.05 for all).

- Summary and Recommendations: A small amount of high-quality evidence supports the use of PRP in chronic refractory patellar tendinopathy and LR-PRP is recommended. Given the small number of studies supporting this conclusion, further clinical trials will help make this suggestion more robust.

Achilles Tendinopathy

In a prospective randomized trial, de Vos and colleagues[46,47] found no significant benefits with LR-PRP versus a saline solution injection as an adjunct to eccentric exercises for mid-Achilles tendinosis. The investigators reported no significant differences in Achilles tendon structure, the degree of neovascularization, and clinical outcome compared with the saline solution group. In a follow-up study on the same patients, de Jonge and colleagues[13] similarly reported no significant benefit in terms of pain reduction, activity level, and tendon appearance on ultrasound at 1 year after injection of PRP for chronic Achilles tendinopathy. A more recent RCT by Boesen and colleagues[12] compared 4 LP-PRP injections each 14 days apart against sham injection with a few drops of subcutaneous saline. All participants performed eccentric Achilles training and the group treated with PRP had significantly improved pain, function, and activity scores at all time points throughout the 6-month follow-up period compared with sham injection. Of note, however, this study also found a comparable improvement with a single high-volume injection (50 mL) of 0.5% bupivacaine (10 mL), methylprednisolone (20 mg), and normal saline (40 mL).

- Summary and Recommendations: Evidence for the use of PRP in Achilles tendinopathy is mixed at best, and therefore routine use of PRP in Achilles tendinopathy is not supported by current literature. As stated, one clinical trial[12] reported efficacy of 4 LP-PRP injections, but also found similar results for high-volume injection of anesthetic, corticosteroid, and saline, perhaps suggesting the benefit may be due to mechanical volume effects.

Rotator Cuff Tendinopathy

Few high-level RCTs have analyzed PRP as a conservative management strategy for rotator cuff pathology. Kesikburun and colleagues[39] looked at subacromial PRP injections in patients with chronic rotator cuff pathology (pain >3 months, with MRI confirming pathology, and >50% relief with subacromial anesthetic injection). The study found no difference in its patient-reported outcome scores when compared with a placebo subacromial injection of saline. In contrast, in an RCT, Rha and colleagues[40] demonstrated significant improvements in pain following 2 injections of LR-PRP 4 weeks apart compared with placebo. Shams and colleagues[41] reported comparable improvements between subacromial PRP and corticosteroid injection in Western Ontario Rotator Cuff Index, Shoulder Pain Disability Index, and VAS shoulder pain with Neer test.

- Summary and Recommendations: Although there remains a paucity of evidence to routinely recommend PRP injections for rotator cuff tendinopathy, PRP may be a safe and effective alternative to corticosteroid injections in conservative treatment of rotator cuff tendinopathy.

Plantar Fasciitis

Several RCTs have evaluated PRP injection in the management of chronic plantar fasciitis. Although the current standard injection therapy following failure of more conservative management has been a local injection of corticosteroid, it often requires multiple injections that can be associated with fat pad atrophy or plantar fascia rupture.[48] The potential of PRP as a local injection treatment mitigates these concerns. Two recent meta-analyses[49,50] evaluated PRP injections against corticosteroid injections, concluding that PRP injections were a viable alternative to corticosteroid injections with respect to efficacy, with some studies demonstrating superiority of PRP.[31–34,36–38] Given the small sample sizes and limited number of high-quality RCTs, larger-scale high-quality RCTs with more extensive follow-up will be warranted.

- Summary and Recommendations: PRP injections are an effective treatment for improving pain and function in chronic plantar fasciitis and may be superior to corticosteroids, especially considering the complications of multiple corticosteroid injections that are not associated with PRP.

OSTEOARTHRITIS

When considering biologic approaches to cartilage pathology, it is important to understand that osteoarthritis (OA) has unique characteristics with respect to joint biology, homeostasis, and levels of metalloproteases and inflammatory cytokines.[51] The idea of using PRP for cartilage regeneration is based on in vitro basic science literature that suggests that growth factors released by the platelet alpha granules may increase the synthetic capacity of chondrocytes through upregulation of gene expression, proteoglycan production, and deposition of type II collagen.[52–54] Clinical reports on the use of PRP for cartilage injury have involved patients with OA of the knee or hip (**Table 3**).

Osteoarthritis of the Knee

There have been a large volume of studies assessing the efficacy of intra-articular PRP injections for OA of the knee. PRP has been compared against placebo, other alternative injections (corticosteroid, hyaluronic acid [HA]), oral medication (Tylenol 500 mg every 8 hours), homeopathic treatments (ozone therapy), and lifestyle changes.[74] Shen and colleagues[75] performed a meta-analysis looking at 14 RCTs comprising 1423 patients. Individual RCTs had different preparations of PRP including LR-PRP, LP-PRP, and plasma rich in growth factor (PRGF) Endoret.[75] The meta-analysis demonstrated that multiple injections of PRP showed significant improvement in Western Ontario and McMaster Universities Osteoarthritis Index (WOMAC) scores at 3-month, 6-month, and 12-month follow-ups when compared with the controls ($P = .02$, .004, $< .001$, respectively), and PRP did not show increased risk of

Table 3
Study design characteristics for PRP versus control injection for osteoarthritis

Indication	Study and Year of Publication	Level of Evidence	Sample Size PRP	Sample Size Control	Type of PRP	Number of Injections	Intervention/Injection Volume and Contents PRP	Intervention/Injection Volume and Contents Control	Follow-up, mo	Favors PRP?
Hip OA	Battaglia et al,[55] 2013	I	50	50	LR-PRP	3	5 mL PRP	30 mg HA	12	−
Hip OA	Dallari et al,[56] 2016	I	44, +HA:31	36	NR	3	7 mL PRP + HA	30 mg HA	12	+
Hip OA	Doria et al,[57] 2017	II	40	40	NR	3	5 mL PRP	15 mg HA	12	−
Hip OA	Sante et al,[58] 2016	I	21	22	NR	3	3 mL PRP	30 mg HA	4	+
Knee OA	Cerza et al,[59] 2012	I	60	60	LP-PRP	4	5.5 mL PRP	20 mg HA	4	+
Knee OA	Cole et al,[60] 2017	I	49	50	LP-PRP	3	4 mL PRP	16 mg HA injection	12	+
Knee OA	Duymus et al,[61] 2017	I	41	HA:40, Ozone:39	NR	2	5 mL PRP	40 mg HA, 15 mL ozone	12	+
Knee OA	Filardo et al,[62] 2015	I	96	96	LR-PRP	3	5 mL PRP	30 mg HA	12	−
Knee OA	Filardo et al,[63] 2012	I	54	55	LR-PRP	3	5 mL PRP	NR HA	12	−
Knee OA	Gormeli et al,[64] 2017	I	PRP(3x):46 PRP(1x):45	HA:46, Placebo:45	NR	3 vs 1	5 mL PRP	30 mg HA, NR saline	6	+
Knee OA	Lana et al,[65] 2016	I	36, +HA: 33	36	NR	3	5 mL PRP + 20 mg HA	20 mg HA	12	+
Knee OA	Montanez et al,[66] 2016	I	28	27	NR	3	NR	NR HA	6	+

Condition	Study		PRP group	Placebo	PRP type	Injections	PRP	Control	Follow-up	Outcome
Knee OA	Patel et al,[67] 2013	—	PRP1:27 PRP2:25	Placebo:26	LP-PRP	1 vs 2	8 mL PRP	8 mL Saline	6	+
Knee OA	Paterson et al,[68] 2016	—	12	11	NR	3	3 mL PRP	3 mL HA	3	–
Knee OA	Raeissadat et al,[69] 2015	—	87	73	LR-PRP	2	4–6 mL PRP	20 mg HA	12	+
Knee OA	Rayegani et al,[70] 2014	—	31	31	LR-PRP	2	4–6 mL PRP + therapeutic exercise	Therapeutic exercise alone	6	+
Knee OA	Sanchez et al,[71] 2012	—	89	87	LP-PRP	3	8 mL PRGF	NR HA	6	+
Knee OA	Simental et al,[72] 2016	—	33	32	LP-PRP	3	3 mL PRP	Tylenol 500 mg q8h	4	+
Knee OA	Smith et al,[73] 2016	—	15	15	LP-PRP	3	3–8 mL PRP	3–8 mL Saline	12	+
Knee OA	Vaquerizao et al,[74] 2013	—	48	48	LP-PRP	3	8 mL PRGF	NR HA	11	+

Abbreviations: HA, hyaluronic acid; LP-PRP, leukocyte-poor PRP; LR-PRP, leukocyte-rich PRP; NR, not reported; OA, osteoarthritis; PRGF, plasma rich in growth factors.

postinjection adverse effects (Relative risk 1.40; 95% confidence interval 0.80–2/40; $I^2 = 59\%$; $P = .24$).[75] They concluded that intra-articular PRP injections are more efficacious in the treatment of knee OA with respect to pain relief and patient-reported outcomes versus other alternative injections.

In the various individual studies within that meta-analysis, it was shown that many subjects who underwent intra-articular injections of PRP reported pain relief compared with baseline. On subgroup analysis examining the efficacy of PRP-based severity of knee OA, PRP was shown more effective in patients with mild to moderate OA.[59,61,64–66,68,69,71] However, a few studies demonstrated no difference in WOMAC scores when compared with HA injection,[60,62,63,67] whereas other studies showed diminishing results in pain relief and function after a certain amount of time.[68] One possible explanation for this discrepancy is the heterogeneity of the PRP preparations and regimens being evaluated for OA of the knee.

A meta-analysis by Riboh and colleagues[76] compared LP-PRP and LR-PRP in the treatment of knee osteoarthritis and found that LP-PRP[59,71] injections resulted in significantly improved WOMAC scores compared with HA or placebo.[67,77] Patel and colleagues[67] performed a prospective randomized trial comparing single-injection or double-injection LP-PRP with saline solution in 78 patients with early OA. They concluded that a single injection of PRP was as effective as a double injection. On the other hand, Filardo and colleagues[62] enrolled 192 patients in a randomized controlled study and found no difference between LR-PRP and HA, providing further evidence that LP-PRP may be an effective choice for treatment of OA symptoms, whereas LR-PRP appears not to be.[76] The biological basis for this may be in the relative level of inflammatory versus anti-inflammatory mediators present in LR-PRP and LP-PRP. Inflammatory mediators TNF-α, IL-6, interferon-γ, and IL-1β are increased significantly in the presence of LR-PRP,[10,78,79] whereas injection of LP-PRP increases IL-4 and IL-10, which are anti-inflammatory mediators. IL-10 specifically was found to be helpful in the treatment of hip OA,[56] and may also suppress the release of the inflammatory mediators TNF-α, IL-6, and IL-1β, and block the inflammatory pathway by neutralizing nuclear factor–kB activity.[10,56,70,72,78] In addition to its deleterious effects on chondrocytes, LR-PRP may also fail to help treat OA symptoms due to its effect on synoviocytes. Braun and colleagues[80] found that treatment of synovial cells with LR-PRP or erythrocytes resulted in significant proinflammatory mediator production and cell death.

- Summary and Recommendations: Intra-articular injection of LP-PRP is a safe treatment option for knee OA, and many RCTs have demonstrated its ability to reduce pain symptoms and increase.[73,75] Larger studies with longer follow-up need to be done to characterize its long-term efficacy.

Osteoarthritis of the Hip

Compared with knee OA, studies on the effects of PRP for hip OA have been limited, with 4 RCTs (to date) comparing PRP injections for OA of the hip with HA injections. Battaglia and colleagues[55] compared clinical efficacy of PRP and HA injections in 100 patients with chronic symptomatic hip OA. Patients were randomized to the 2 groups, and VAS and Harris Hip Score (HHS) outcomes were measured at baseline and at 1, 3, 6, and 12 months. Both PRP and HA injections demonstrated significant improvement at all time points with peak improvement at 3 months, and gradual diminishing effects thereafter to 12 months. The outcome scores at 12 months still displayed significant improvement when compared with baseline ($P<.0005$)[55]; however, there was no statistically significant difference between PRP and HA treatment groups.

Di Sante and colleagues[58] looked at 43 patients with severe hip OA who were randomized to receive either an intra-articular PRP injection or an intra-articular HA injection. Outcomes were measured using the VAS and WOMAC pain scores at baseline, 4 weeks, and 16 weeks following treatment. In the PRP group, VAS scores significantly decreased at 4 weeks but not at 16, suggesting an initial, but not sustained reduction in pain. Interestingly, the HA group saw a significant difference at week 16, but not week 4 when compared with baseline.[58]

Dallari and colleagues[56] evaluated PRP against HA injections for hip OA, and also compared the combination of HA and PRP injected together to both injections alone. The PRP group was found to have the lowest VAS score of all 3 groups at all follow-up periods (2 months, 6 months, and 12 month). The PRP group also had a significantly better WOMAC score at 2 and 6 months, but not at 12 months. In a different study, Doria and colleagues[57] performed a double-blind RCT comparing patients who received 3 consecutive weekly injections of PRP versus 3 HA injections. The study showed no significant difference between the PRP and HA groups, but both groups showed improved HHS, WOMAC, and VAS scores at 6 and 12 months following treatment. None of the studies showed an adverse effect from intra-articular PRP injections into the hip and all concluded that PRP was safe.

Overall, although limited data, intra-articular injection of PRP for hip OA has been shown to be safe and have some efficacy in pain reduction and function as measured by patient-reported outcome scores. Multiple studies have shown PRP to initially have a better pain reduction when compared with HA; however, that initial advantage seems to decrease over time with PRP and HA having very similar efficacy by 12 months.

- Summary and Recommendations: PRP may have some efficacy for early and temporal pain relief in hip OA and overall had very similar efficacy as HA injections. As there have been a small number of clinical studies evaluating the use of PRP for OA of the hip, more level I evidence is needed to determine if PRP can be used as an alternative conservative treatment to delay surgery for OA of the hip.

SURGICAL AUGMENTATION
Rotator Cuff Repair

Several high-level clinical studies have evaluated the use of PRP products as augmentations in arthroscopic repair of rotator cuff tears (**Table 4**). Many of the studies have specifically analyzed the use of platelet-rich fibrin matrix preparation for augmentation (PRFM),[81,82,90,91,93] whereas other studies analyzed the use of injected PRP directly into the repair site.[87,89,94] There is, however, significant heterogeneity of the PRP or PRFM preparations in these studies. Results were obtained with patient-directed outcomes, most commonly University of California–Los Angeles (UCLA), American Shoulder and Elbow Society (ASES) and Constant Shoulder scores, Simple Shoulder Test (SST) scores, and VAS pain scores. Some studies have also used imaging, such as ultrasound and MRI, to measure differences in tendon healing, healing time, and retear rates. Objective clinical data, such as rotator cuff strength and shoulder range of motion (ROM) have also been collected to measure functional outcome differences.[39,84,86,87,91] Most of the data have shown little utility for PRP in rotator cuff tendinopathy or as augmentation in arthroscopic rotator cuff repair.[39,82,83,86,88–91,93,95,96] However, limited data have shown some effect in reducing perioperative pain.[41,86,89,95]

Saltzman and colleagues[97] and Filardo and colleagues[98] performed large meta-analyses, and showed that PRP had no significant benefit in augmentation of

Table 4
Study design characteristics of surgical augmentation with PRP in rotator cuff repair

Indication	Study and Year of Publication	Level of Evidence	Sample Size		Type of PRP	Number of Injections	Intervention/Injection Volume and Contents		Follow-up, mo	Favors PRP?
			PRP	Control			PRP	Control		
Rotator cuff repair	Bergeson et al,[81] 2012	III	16	21	PRFM	1	PRFM + single-row or double-row repair	Single-row or double-row repair	12	−
Rotator cuff repair	Castricini et al,[82] 2011	I	43	45	NR-PRFM	1	PRFM + double-row repair	Double-row repair	16	−
Rotator cuff repair	D'Ambrosi et al,[83] 2016	I	20	20	NR	1	16 mL PRP + single-row repair	Single-row repair	6	+
Rotator cuff repair	Ebert et al,[84] 2017	I	30	30	LP-PRP	2 (day 7 and 14)	2–4 mL PRP + double-row repair	Double-row repair	42	+
Rotator cuff repair	Gumina et al,[85] 2012	I	39	37	LR-PRFM	1	PRFM + single-row repair	Single-row repair	12	−
Rotator cuff repair	Holtby et al,[86] 2016	I	41	41	LP-PRP	1	7 mL PRP + single-row repair	Single-row repair	6	−
Rotator cuff repair	Jo et al,[87] 2015	I	37	37	LP-PRP	3	3 mL PRP gel + double-row repair	Double-row repair	12	+
Rotator cuff repair	Malavolta et al,[88] 2014	I	27	27	LR-PRP	1	20 mL PRP + single-row repair	Single-row repair	24	−
Rotator cuff repair	Randelli et al,[89] 2011	I	26	27	LR-PRP	1	6 mL PRP + single-row repair	Single-row repair	24	+
Rotator cuff repair	Rodeo et al,[90] 2012	II	40	39	PRFM	1	PRFM + single-row or double-row repair	Single-row or double-row repair	12	−
Rotator cuff repair	Weber et al,[91] 2013	I	30	30	LP-PRFM	1	PRFM clot + single-row repair	Single-row repair	12	−
Rotator cuff repair	Zumstein et al,[92] 2016	I	17	18	LR-PRFM	1	PRFM + double-row repair	Double-row repair	12	−

Abbreviations: LP-PRP, leukocyte-poor PRP; LR-PRP, leukocyte-rich PRP; NR, not reported; PRFM, platelet-rich fibrin matrix. +, indicates that the trial found in favor of PRP; −, indicates the trial did not favor of PRP.

arthroscopically repaired rotator cuffs. Saltzman and colleagues[97] looked at 7 meta-analyses encompassing a total of 3193 patients. At mean follow-up of 12 to 21 months, no significant difference was found when compared with controls in 5 of 6 studies measuring constant scores, 6 of 6 measuring UCLA scores, 4 of 5 measuring ASES scores, and 3 of 5 measuring SST scores. However, a subgroup analysis did see a trend toward better outcomes with PRP in the form of PRFM; in the treatment of small and medium tears versus large/massive tears; when applied to the tendon-bone interface versus over the tendon; and when applied with double-row versus single-row rotator cuff repairs.[97]

Vavken and colleagues[99] performed a meta-analysis of 14 studies looking at PRP-augmented rotator cuff repairs. They were divided into subgroups of small and medium tears (<3 cm) and large tears (>3 cm). In large tears, there were no beneficial effects of PRP-augmented surgery. In small and medium tears, there was a beneficial effect of reducing retear rates ($P = .038$).

Some individual studies have determined a utility for PRP in different tear sizes and patterns. Cai and colleagues[96] found PRP augmentation to be associated with a lower failure to heal rate in small to moderate tears. Jo and colleagues[87] found that PRP application with medium and large tear repairs led to a decrease in retear rates (3% vs 20% in the conventional group) and an increased cross-sectional area of the supraspinatus on follow-up MRI when compared with no augmentation. Potentially due to the anti-inflammatory properties of PRP, PRP application has been shown to reduce pain in the early postoperative period following surgery.[83,86,89] Flury and colleagues[95] showed similar pain reduction when compared with an injection of ropivacaine.

- Summary and Recommendations: Evidence from randomized clinical trials and large meta-analyses do not demonstrate an absolute benefit of PRP augmentation in rotator cuff repair surgery. A recent critical analysis review[100] reached a similar conclusion that PRP could not be routinely recommended as an augmentation in rotator cuff repair, but that activated PRFM delivered at the bone-tendon interface in conjunction with double-row repair technique had the best results in subgroup analyses. Some limited data have shown PRP may be useful in reducing postoperative pain and repair of small and medium tears.

Achilles Tendon Repair

The effects of PRP to augment healing in Achilles tendon ruptures have been promising in preclinical models. Most studies in rodents show a beneficial effect of platelets on the healing of acute Achilles tendon ruptures when used as an adjunctive therapy.[101–108] Caution is warranted, however, when extrapolating results from preclinical Achilles rupture models to human patients,[109] due to the difference in the size of the tendons between species, which has significant effects in terms of diffusion and cellular migration distances.[110] Furthermore, rodents tend to load their healing Achilles tendons to a greater extent than humans, which leads to more favorable biomechanical outcomes.[111]

Clinical trials in humans are limited with respect to the use of PRP in the repair of acute Achilles tendon tears, and their findings are somewhat conflicting. Schepull and colleagues[112] evaluated the use of PRP in Achilles tendon repair in a randomized study (n = 30) in which PRP was injected into the injury site at the time of primary suture repair. Although no differences were reported with regard to tendon elasticity and heel raise index between the PRP and control groups, the investigators did note a lower Achilles Tendon Total Rupture score among the PRP group, which suggests a detrimental effect of PRP on subjective outcome after repair. Additionally, another study also demonstrated equivalence in structural and functional results in patients with Achilles tendon ruptures surgically treated with and without addition of PRP.[113] However, Zou and colleagues[114] enrolled 36 patients with acute Achilles tendon rupture in a prospective randomized controlled study using intraoperative LR-PRP injection versus repair without PRP. Patients were followed for 24 months. Patients from the PRP group had better isokinetic muscle at 3 months and had higher SF-36 and Leppilahti scores at 6 and 12 months, respectively ($P<.05$ for all). Ankle ROM was also significantly better in the PRP group at all time points of 6, 12, and 24 months ($P<.001$).

- Summary and Recommendations: Injection of PRP is not definitively beneficial as a surgical augmentation for acute Achilles tendon repair, although the available literature is conflicting.

Anterior Cruciate Ligament Surgery

The success of anterior cruciate ligament (ACL) surgery not only hinges on technical factors (eg, graft-tunnel placement and graft fixation) but also biologic healing of the ACL graft. Studies on the use of PRP in ACL reconstruction surgery have focused on 3 biologic processes: (1) osteoligamentous integration of the graft into the tibial and femoral tunnels, (2) maturation of the articular portion of the graft, (3) and graft harvest site healing and pain reduction.[115] Within the literature, ACL graft maturation tends to be assessed with MRI. The assumption is that a low homogeneous intensity signal on T2-weighted and proton density–weighted MRI is likely indicative of a healthy maturing ACL graft. In terms of the effect of PRP on ACL graft maturation, some studies have demonstrated improved graft maturation with PRP,[116–119] whereas others report no significant differences.[120,121] The investigators of a recent systematic review of 11 controlled trials, which included studies in which statistical significance was not reached, concluded that PRP likely improves ACL graft maturation by up to 50%. The investigators pointed to insufficient sample size as a potential rationale for lack of statistical significance despite MRI improvement in some metrics measuring ACL graft maturation.[122]

The other component to successful biologic healing of an ACL graft is graft–bone tunnel incorporation. Recent data on the use of PRP to augment healing of the graft-bone interface has shown no clinical benefit of PRP in tunnel widening or osteointegration of the graft.[120,123] Vogrin and colleagues[121] evaluated the effects of PRP gel treatment for hamstring autograft ACL reconstruction in a controlled, double-blind study. The investigators reported MRI evidence of improved vascularization along the ACL graft-bone interface at 3 months with use of PRP, but the observed benefit dissipated by 6 months after surgery. Other studies have similarly reported limited to no evidence to support the use of PRP to augment ACL graft–bone tunnel incorporation.[116,124] Of note is that nearly all of the studies used an LR-PRP formulation, and LR-PRP formulations increase local tissue inflammation, which may delay or alter healing.[8]

One final point of consideration is whether any of the observed benefit of PRP on ACL graft maturation or graft-tunnel healing would translate into improved clinical results. The best available evidence seems to suggest no significant benefit for functional outcomes with PRP augmentation.[116,120,125] Ventura and colleagues[125] found no differences in knee injury and osteoarthritis outcome score (KOOS) scores, Tegner scores, or KT-1000 measurements between the PRP-treated group and control subjects at 6 months after surgery, despite reporting a significant difference in graft appearance. Orrego and colleagues[116] similarly noted no significant benefit in both Lysholm and International Knee Documentation Committee (IKDC) scores at 6 months after surgery, despite identifying a positive effect of PRP on graft maturation. Current literature suggests that PRP may improve the rate at which ACL grafts achieve a low signal on MRI T2-weighted imaging, but likely has little to no effect on graft-tunnel incorporation. A demonstrable benefit in patient outcome after use of PRP in patients undergoing ACL surgery is also lacking.

Other clinical trials have assessed the impact of PRP on donor site (graft harvest site) pain and healing, with some promising early results. De Almeida and colleagues[126] looked at adding PRP to the patellar tendon harvest site and measuring patient-reported pain scores and patellar tending gapping on MRI at 6 months following surgery. The investigators found that patients reported better immediate postoperative pain scores, and at 6 months there was significantly less gapping on MRI, although isokinetic testing results were no different.[126] Seijas and colleagues[127] looked at anterior knee pain after bone-patellar-bone autograft ACL reconstruction with PRP application, and found decreased anterior knee pain when compared with controls. In a different study, Cervellin and colleagues[128] did not see a significant difference in VAS pain scores, but found that the PRP group had a significantly higher VISA score.

- Summary and Recommendations: More studies are needed to investigate the effect of PRP on ACL graft integration, maturation, and donor site pain. Early studies have shown no significant clinical effect of PRP on graft integration or maturation, but newer studies have shown promising results in decreasing donor site pain.

ANKLE SPRAINS

There are very little high-level data analyzing PRP injections in ankle sprains, with (to date) 2 published RCTs available. Rowden and colleagues[129] performed a double-blinded placebo-controlled randomized clinical trial of patients with acute ankle sprains in the emergency room comparing ultrasound-guided LR-PRP injections with local anesthetic versus injection of normal saline with local anesthetic. Injections were performed adjacent to an injured ligament if visualized on ultrasound or otherwise were injected into the site of maximal tenderness. For all patients, a posterior splint was placed with non–weight-bearing restrictions for 3 days. Pain medication was given at the physician's discretion. Primary outcome measures were VAS pain score and Lower Extremity Functional Sale (LEFS) on day 0 (baseline), day 3, and day 8. The investigators found that there was no statistical difference in the VAS pain score or LEFS between the 2 groups.[1] Laver and colleagues[130] randomized 16 elite athletes diagnosed with high ankle sprains, including an injured anteroinferior tibiofibular ligament to treatment with either an ultrasound-guided LP-PRP injection at initial presentation with a repeat injection 7 days later in conjunction with a rehabilitation program, versus rehabilitation program alone. Primary outcomes were measured by return-to-play and dynamic imaging studies. All patients received the same rehabilitation protocol and return-to-play criteria. The study found the LP-PRP group returned to play in a shorter amount of time (40.8 days) compared with the control (59.6 days, $P<.006$).[130] Only 1 patient had residual pain after return to play in the PRP group, whereas 5 patients had residual pain in the control. No significant difference was seen in the dynamic imaging studies in external rotation between the 2 groups 6 weeks post injury.

- Summary and Recommendations: PRP has not been shown to be efficacious in the setting of acute ankle sprains, but limited evidence suggests that LP-PRP injections may be helpful in high ankle sprains to reduce return-to-play time and decrease incidence of residual pain in elite athletes. However, due to the limited amount of high-level evidence, the use of PRP injections cannot be routinely recommended for high ankle sprains.

MUSCLE INJURIES

The use of PRP in the treatment of muscle injuries has attracted a significant amount of interest in recent years. Similar to tendon healing, the steps in muscle healing involve the initial inflammatory response, which is followed by cell proliferation, differentiation, and tissue remodeling. Hamid and colleagues[131] conducted a single-blind randomized study of 28 patients with grade 2 hamstring muscle injuries comparing an injection of LR-PRP with a rehabilitation program, versus rehabilitation alone. The group treated with LR-PRP was able to return to play in a significantly shorter amount of time compared with controls (average 26.7 vs 42.5 days, $P = .02$), but structural improvement was not achieved. In a double-blind RCT, Reurink and colleagues[132] evaluated 80 patients comparing intramuscular PRP injections for the treatment of acute hamstring muscle injuries as diagnosed on MRI with placebo saline injections, with all patients receiving standard rehabilitation. The patients were followed for 6 months, and the investigators reported no significant differences between the groups in return-to-play time or in reinjury rates.

Although clinical studies have not found PRP to be efficacious in treating muscle injuries, basic science research may lead to an improved understanding of treatment modalities. In vitro work has found that PRP is capable of leading to myoblast proliferation, but not to myoblast differentiation,[133] a requisite step in producing muscle tissue. Furthermore, growth factors contained in platelets, specifically myostatin and TGF-β1, are actually detrimental to muscle regeneration.[134,135] Miroshnychenko and colleagues[136] found in vitro that treatment with PPP or PRP with a second spin to remove the platelets induced myoblasts into muscle differentiation. This suggests that perhaps the most beneficial treatment of muscle injuries may be with PPP, although in vivo animal studies followed by human clinical trials will be necessary to further explore this treatment option in the future.

- Summary and Recommendations: PRP injections have not been found to be an efficacious treatment modality in the treatment of muscle injuries in current clinical studies, but preclinical studies suggest that perhaps future clinical investigation into the use of PPP or PRP with platelets removed may be beneficial.

FRACTURE AND NONUNION MANAGEMENT

Most preclinical investigations favor the use of PRP to improve bone healing.[137,138] This is mainly due to accelerated and increased bone regeneration demonstrated in fracture models treated with PRP.[139–146] Additionally, PRP treatment has been shown to ameliorate bone strength in a rodent osteotomy model.[144] In isolation, however, PRP treatment alone does not effectively heal critical-sized bone defects.[147–149]

Despite the positive findings in the preclinical literature, there is no consensus to support the routine use of PRP to enhance bone healing based on high-quality clinical studies. To this point, a recent review of PRP and acute fracture treatment notes that 3 of the included RCTs failed to show benefit with respect to functional outcomes, whereas 2 of the included studies showed superior clinical outcomes.[138] Most trials in this review (6 of 8) studied efficacy of PRP when combined with other biologics, such as mesenchymal stem cells and/or bone graft, to promote fracture healing. In terms of nonunion treatment, there was only 1 RCT identified reporting clinical outcomes measures. This study failed to show a benefit of PRP when compared with bone morphogenetic protein 7 (which is standard of care) when treating tibia nonunions.[150]

- Summary and Recommendations: Current evidence does not support the use of PRP in acute fracture or nonunion management

SUMMARY OF RECOMMENDATIONS

PRP remains a promising treatment for musculoskeletal maladies, and clinical data to date have shown that PRP is safe. However, evidence of its efficacy has been mixed and highly variable depending on the specific indication. Additional future high-quality large clinical trials will be critical in shaping our perspective of this treatment option. The heterogeneity of PRP preparations, both presently and historically, leads sweeping recommendations about its utility impossible to make. This heterogeneity has also made interpreting existing literature more complicated. Nonetheless, based on the current best available literature, the following recommendations are summarized:

- There is abundant high-quality level I evidence to recommend LR-PRP injections for lateral epicondylitis and LP-PRP injections for OA of the knee
- There is a moderate amount of high-quality level I evidence to recommend LR-PRP injections for patellar tendinopathy and PRP injections for plantar fasciitis
- There is currently insufficient high-quality evidence for recommendation, but small clinical trials have shown promising efficacy for PRP injections for rotator cuff tendinopathy, OA of the hip, donor site pain in ACL reconstruction with patellar tendon autograft, and LP-PRP injections for high ankle sprains
- The best available clinical evidence does not demonstrate efficacy of PRP injections for Achilles tendinopathy, acute fracture, or nonunion; surgical augmentation with PRP in rotator cuff repair, Achilles tendon repair, and ACL reconstruction; and efficacy has not been shown with PRP injections for muscle injuries, although preclinical studies suggest PPP may hold promise for muscle injuries but clinical trials will be necessary to validate this.

REFERENCES

1. Boswell SG, Cole BJ, Sundman EA, et al. Platelet-rich plasma: a milieu of bioactive factors. Arthroscopy 2012;28(3):429–39.
2. Foster TE, Puskas BL, Mandelbaum BR, et al. Platelet-rich plasma: from basic science to clinical applications. Am J Sports Med 2009;37(11):2259–72.
3. Le A, Dragoo JL. Orthobiologics: clinical application of platelet-rich plasma and stem cell therapy. In: DeLee & Drez's orthopaedic sports medicine. 5th edition. Elsevier; in press.
4. Marx RE. Platelet-rich plasma (PRP): what is PRP and what is not PRP? Implant Dent 2001;10(4):225–8.
5. Degen RM, Bernard JA, Oliver KS, et al. Commercial separation systems designed for preparation of platelet-rich plasma yield differences in cellular composition. HSS J 2017;13(1):75–80.
6. Magalon J, Bausset O, Serratrice N, et al. Characterization and comparison of 5 platelet-rich plasma preparations in a single-donor model. Arthroscopy 2014; 30(5):629–38.
7. Castillo TN, Pouliot MA, Kim HJ, et al. Comparison of growth factor and platelet concentration from commercial platelet-rich plasma separation systems. Am J Sports Med 2011;39(2):266–71.
8. Dragoo JL, Braun HJ, Durham JL, et al. Comparison of the acute inflammatory response of two commercial platelet-rich plasma systems in healthy rabbit tendons. Am J Sports Med 2012;40(6):1274–81.
9. Mazzocca AD, McCarthy MBR, Chowaniec DM, et al. Platelet-rich plasma differs according to preparation method and human variability. J Bone Joint Surg Am 2012;94(4):308–16.

10. Sundman EA, Cole BJ, Fortier LA. Growth factor and catabolic cytokine concentrations are influenced by the cellular composition of platelet-rich plasma. Am J Sports Med 2011;39(10):2135–40.

11. McCarrel T, Fortier L. Temporal growth factor release from platelet-rich plasma, trehalose lyophilized platelets, and bone marrow aspirate and their effect on tendon and ligament gene expression. J Orthop Res 2009;27(8):1033–42.

12. Boesen AP, Hansen R, Boesen MI, et al. Effect of high-volume injection, platelet-rich plasma, and sham treatment in chronic midportion Achilles tendinopathy: a randomized double-blinded prospective study. Am J Sports Med 2017;45(9):2034–43.

13. de Jonge S, de Vos RJ, Weir A, et al. One-year follow-up of platelet-rich plasma treatment in chronic Achilles tendinopathy: a double-blind randomized placebo-controlled trial. Am J Sports Med 2011;39(8):1623–9.

14. Krogh TP, Ellingsen T, Christensen R, et al. Ultrasound-guided injection therapy of Achilles tendinopathy with platelet-rich plasma or saline: a randomized, blinded, placebo-controlled trial. Am J Sports Med 2016;44(8):1990–7.

15. Behera P, Dhillon M, Aggarwal S, et al. Leukocyte-poor platelet-rich plasma versus bupivacaine for recalcitrant lateral epicondylar tendinopathy. J Orthop Surg 2015;23(1):6–10.

16. Gautam V, Verma S, Batra S, et al. Platelet-rich plasma versus corticosteroid injection for recalcitrant lateral epicondylitis: clinical and ultrasonographic evaluation. J Orthop Surg 2015;23(1):1–5.

17. Gosens T, Peerbooms JC, van Laar W, et al. Ongoing positive effect of platelet-rich plasma versus corticosteroid injection in lateral epicondylitis: a double-blind randomized controlled trial with 2-year follow-up. Am J Sports Med 2011;39(6):1200–8.

18. Krogh TP, Fredberg U, Stengaard-Pedersen K, et al. Treatment of lateral epicondylitis with platelet-rich plasma, glucocorticoid, or saline: a randomized, double-blind, placebo-controlled trial. Am J Sports Med 2013;41(3):625–35.

19. Lebiedziński R, Synder M, Buchcic P, et al. A randomized study of autologous conditioned plasma and steroid injections in the treatment of lateral epicondylitis. Int Orthop 2015;39(11):2199–203.

20. Mishra AK, Skrepnik NV, Edwards SG, et al. Efficacy of platelet-rich plasma for chronic tennis elbow: a double-blind, prospective, multicenter, randomized controlled trial of 230 patients. Am J Sports Med 2014;42(2):463–71.

21. Montalvan B, Le Goux P, Klouche S, et al. Inefficacy of ultrasound-guided local injections of autologous conditioned plasma for recent epicondylitis: results of a double-blind placebo-controlled randomized clinical trial with one-year follow-up. Rheumatology 2016;55(2):279–85.

22. Palacio EP, Schiavetti RR, Kanematsu M, et al. Effects of platelet-rich plasma on lateral epicondylitis of the elbow: prospective randomized controlled trial. Rev Bras Ortop 2016;51(1):90–5.

23. Stenhouse G, Sookur P, Watson M. Do blood growth factors offer additional benefit in refractory lateral epicondylitis? A prospective, randomized pilot trial of dry needling as a stand-alone procedure versus dry needling and autologous conditioned plasma. Skeletal Radiol 2013;42(11):1515–20.

24. Yadav R. Comparison of local injection of platelet rich plasma and corticosteroids in the treatment of lateral epicondylitis of humerus. J Clin Diagn Res 2015;9(7):RC05–7.

25. Dragoo JL, Wasterlain AS, Braun HJ, et al. Platelet-rich plasma as a treatment for patellar tendinopathy: a double-blind, randomized controlled trial. Am J Sports Med 2014;42(3):610–8.
26. Vetrano M, Castorina A, Vulpiani MC, et al. Platelet-rich plasma versus focused shock waves in the treatment of jumper's knee in athletes. Am J Sports Med 2013;41(4):795–803.
27. Acosta-Olivo C, Elizondo-Rodriguez J, Lopez-Cavazos R, et al. Plantar fasciitis—a comparison of treatment with intralesional steroids versus platelet-rich plasma randomized, blinded study. J Am Podiatr Med Assoc 2017;107(6): 490–6.
28. Akşahin E, Doğruyol D, Yüksel HY, et al. The comparison of the effect of corticosteroids and platelet-rich plasma (PRP) for the treatment of plantar fasciitis. Arch Orthop Trauma Surg 2012;132(6):781–5.
29. Jain K, Murphy PN, Clough TM. Platelet rich plasma versus corticosteroid injection for plantar fasciitis: a comparative study. Foot 2015;25(4):235–7.
30. Jain SK, Suprashant K, Kumar S, et al. Comparison of plantar fasciitis injected with platelet-rich plasma vs corticosteroids. Foot Ankle Int 2018;39(7):780–6.
31. Mahindra P, Yamin M, Selhi HS, et al. Chronic plantar fasciitis: effect of platelet-rich plasma, corticosteroid, and placebo. Orthopedics 2016;39(2):e285–9.
32. Monto RR. Platelet-rich plasma efficacy versus corticosteroid injection treatment for chronic severe plantar fasciitis. Foot Ankle Int 2014;35(4):313–8.
33. Omar AS, Ibrahim ME, Ahmed AS, et al. Local injection of autologous platelet rich plasma and corticosteroid in treatment of lateral epicondylitis and plantar fasciitis: randomized clinical trial. Egypt Rheumatol 2012;34(2):43–9.
34. Say F, Gürler D, İnkaya E, et al. Comparison of platelet-rich plasma and steroid injection in the treatment of plantar fasciitis. Acta Orthop Traumatol Turc 2014; 48(6):667–72.
35. Sherpy NA, Hammad MA, Hagrass HA, et al. Local injection of autologous platelet rich plasma compared to corticosteroid treatment of chronic plantar fasciitis patients: a clinical and ultrasonographic follow-up study. Egypt Rheumatol 2016;38(3):247–52.
36. Shetty VD, Dhillon M, Hegde C, et al. A study to compare the efficacy of corticosteroid therapy with platelet-rich plasma therapy in recalcitrant plantar fasciitis: a preliminary report. Foot Ankle Surg 2014;20(1):10–3.
37. Tiwari M, Bhargava R. Platelet rich plasma therapy: a comparative effective therapy with promising results in plantar fasciitis. J Clin Orthop Trauma 2013;4(1): 31–5.
38. Vahdatpour B, Kianimehr L, Moradi A, et al. Beneficial effects of platelet-rich plasma on improvement of pain severity and physical disability in patients with plantar fasciitis: a randomized trial. Adv Biomed Res 2016;5:179.
39. Kesikburun S, Tan AK, Yılmaz B, et al. Platelet-rich plasma injections in the treatment of chronic rotator cuff tendinopathy: a randomized controlled trial with 1-year follow-up. Am J Sports Med 2013;41(11):2609–16.
40. Rha D, Park G-Y, Kim Y-K, et al. Comparison of the therapeutic effects of ultrasound-guided platelet-rich plasma injection and dry needling in rotator cuff disease: a randomized controlled trial. Clin Rehabil 2013;27(2):113–22.
41. Shams A, El-Sayed M, Gamal O, et al. Subacromial injection of autologous platelet-rich plasma versus corticosteroid for the treatment of symptomatic partial rotator cuff tears. Eur J Orthop Surg Traumatol 2016;26(8):837–42.
42. Miller LE, Parrish WR, Roides B, et al. Efficacy of platelet-rich plasma injections for symptomatic tendinopathy: systematic review and meta-analysis of

randomised injection-controlled trials. BMJ Open Sport Exerc Med 2017;3(1): e000237.

43. Peerbooms JC, Sluimer J, Bruijn DJ, et al. Positive effect of an autologous platelet concentrate in lateral epicondylitis in a double-blind randomized controlled trial: platelet-rich plasma versus corticosteroid injection with a 1-year follow-up. Am J Sports Med 2010;38(2):255–62.

44. Arirachakaran A, Sukthuayat A, Sisayanarane T, et al. Platelet-rich plasma versus autologous blood versus steroid injection in lateral epicondylitis: systematic review and network meta-analysis. J Orthop Traumatol 2016;17(2):101–12.

45. Krogh TP, Bartels EM, Ellingsen T, et al. Comparative effectiveness of injection therapies in lateral epicondylitis: a systematic review and network meta-analysis of randomized controlled trials. Am J Sports Med 2013;41(6):1435–46.

46. de Vos RJ, Weir A, van Schie HTM, et al. Platelet-rich plasma injection for chronic Achilles tendinopathy: a randomized controlled trial. JAMA 2010; 303(2):144–9.

47. de Vos RJ, Weir A, Tol JL, et al. No effects of PRP on ultrasonographic tendon structure and neovascularisation in chronic midportion Achilles tendinopathy. Br J Sports Med 2011;45(5):387–92.

48. Neufeld SK, Cerrato R. Plantar fasciitis: evaluation and treatment. J Am Acad Orthop Surg 2008;16(6):338–46.

49. Yang W-Y, Han Y-H, Cao X-W, et al. Platelet-rich plasma as a treatment for plantar fasciitis: a meta-analysis of randomized controlled trials. Medicine (Baltimore) 2017;96(44):e8475.

50. Singh P, Madanipour S, Bhamra JS, et al. A systematic review and meta-analysis of platelet-rich plasma versus corticosteroid injections for plantar fasciopathy. Int Orthop 2017;41(6):1169–81.

51. Pearle AD, Warren RF, Rodeo SA. Basic science of articular cartilage and osteoarthritis. Clin Sports Med 2005;24(1):1–12.

52. Spreafico A, Chellini F, Frediani B, et al. Biochemical investigation of the effects of human platelet releasates on human articular chondrocytes. J Cell Biochem 2009;108(5):1153–65.

53. Sun Y, Feng Y, Zhang CQ, et al. The regenerative effect of platelet-rich plasma on healing in large osteochondral defects. Int Orthop 2010;34(4):589–97.

54. Smyth NA, Murawski CD, Fortier LA, et al. Platelet-rich plasma in the pathologic processes of cartilage: review of basic science evidence. Arthroscopy 2013; 29(8):1399–409.

55. Battaglia M, Guaraldi F, Vannini F, et al. Efficacy of ultrasound-guided intra-articular injections of platelet-rich plasma versus hyaluronic acid for hip osteoarthritis. Orthopedics 2013;36(12):e1501–8.

56. Dallari D, Stagni C, Rani N, et al. Ultrasound-guided injection of platelet-rich plasma and hyaluronic acid, separately and in combination, for hip osteoarthritis: a randomized controlled study. Am J Sports Med 2016;44(3):664–71.

57. Doria C, Mosele GR, Caggiari G, et al. Treatment of early hip osteoarthritis: ultrasound-guided platelet rich plasma versus hyaluronic acid injections in a randomized clinical trial. Joints 2017;5(3):152–5.

58. Sante LD, Villani C, Santilli V, et al. Intra-articular hyaluronic acid vs platelet-rich plasma in the treatment of hip osteoarthritis. Med Ultrason 2016;18(4):463–8.

59. Cerza F, Carnì S, Carcangiu A, et al. Comparison between hyaluronic acid and platelet-rich plasma, intra-articular infiltration in the treatment of gonarthrosis. Am J Sports Med 2012;40(12):2822–7.

60. Cole BJ, Karas V, Hussey K, et al. Hyaluronic acid versus platelet-rich plasma: a prospective, double-blind randomized controlled trial comparing clinical outcomes and effects on intra-articular biology for the treatment of knee osteoarthritis. Am J Sports Med 2017;45(2):339–46.

61. Duymus TM, Mutlu S, Dernek B, et al. Choice of intra-articular injection in treatment of knee osteoarthritis: platelet-rich plasma, hyaluronic acid or ozone options. Knee Surg Sports Traumatol Arthrosc 2017;25(2):485–92.

62. Filardo G, Di Matteo B, Di Martino A, et al. Platelet-rich plasma intra-articular knee injections show no superiority versus viscosupplementation: a randomized controlled trial. Am J Sports Med 2015;43(7):1575–82.

63. Filardo G, Kon E, Di Martino A, et al. Platelet-rich plasma vs hyaluronic acid to treat knee degenerative pathology: study design and preliminary results of a randomized controlled trial. BMC Musculoskelet Disord 2012;13:229.

64. Görmeli G, Görmeli CA, Ataoglu B, et al. Multiple PRP injections are more effective than single injections and hyaluronic acid in knees with early osteoarthritis: a randomized, double-blind, placebo-controlled trial. Knee Surg Sports Traumatol Arthrosc 2017;25(3):958–65.

65. Lana JFSD, Weglein A, Sampson SE, et al. Randomized controlled trial comparing hyaluronic acid, platelet-rich plasma and the combination of both in the treatment of mild and moderate osteoarthritis of the knee. J Stem Cells Regen Med 2016;12(2):69–78.

66. Montañez-Heredia E, Irízar S, Huertas PJ, et al. Intra-articular injections of platelet-rich plasma versus hyaluronic acid in the treatment of osteoarthritic knee pain: a randomized clinical trial in the context of the Spanish National Health Care System. Int J Mol Sci 2016;17(7) [pii:E1064].

67. Patel S, Dhillon MS, Aggarwal S, et al. Treatment with platelet-rich plasma is more effective than placebo for knee osteoarthritis: a prospective, double-blind, randomized trial. Am J Sports Med 2013;41(2):356–64.

68. Paterson KL, Nicholls M, Bennell KL, et al. Intra-articular injection of photo-activated platelet-rich plasma in patients with knee osteoarthritis: a double-blind, randomized controlled pilot study. BMC Musculoskelet Disord 2016; 17:67.

69. Raeissadat SA, Rayegani SM, Hassanabadi H, et al. Knee osteoarthritis injection choices: Platelet-Rich Plasma (PRP) versus hyaluronic acid (a one-year randomized clinical trial). Clin Med Insights Arthritis Musculoskelet Disord 2015;8: 1–8.

70. Rayegani SM, Raeissadat SA, Taheri MS, et al. Does intra articular platelet rich plasma injection improve function, pain and quality of life in patients with osteoarthritis of the knee? A randomized clinical trial. Orthop Rev 2014;6(3):5405.

71. Sánchez M, Fiz N, Azofra J, et al. A randomized clinical trial evaluating plasma rich in growth factors (PRGF-Endoret) versus hyaluronic acid in the short-term treatment of symptomatic knee osteoarthritis. Arthroscopy 2012;28(8):1070–8.

72. Simental-Mendía M, Vílchez-Cavazos JF, Peña-Martínez VM, et al. Leukocyte-poor platelet-rich plasma is more effective than the conventional therapy with acetaminophen for the treatment of early knee osteoarthritis. Arch Orthop Trauma Surg 2016;136(12):1723–32.

73. Smith PA. Intra-articular autologous conditioned plasma injections provide safe and efficacious treatment for knee osteoarthritis: an FDA-sanctioned, randomized, double-blind, placebo-controlled clinical trial. Am J Sports Med 2016; 44(4):884–91.

74. Vaquerizo V, Plasencia MÁ, Arribas I, et al. Comparison of intra-articular injections of Plasma Rich in Growth Factors (PRGF-Endoret) versus durolane hyaluronic acid in the treatment of patients with symptomatic osteoarthritis: a randomized controlled trial. Arthroscopy 2013;29(10):1635–43.

75. Shen L, Yuan T, Chen S, et al. The temporal effect of platelet-rich plasma on pain and physical function in the treatment of knee osteoarthritis: systematic review and meta-analysis of randomized controlled trials. J Orthop Surg 2017;12(1):16.

76. Riboh JC, Saltzman BM, Yanke AB, et al. Effect of leukocyte concentration on the efficacy of platelet-rich plasma in the treatment of knee osteoarthritis. Am J Sports Med 2016;44(3):792–800.

77. Hart R, Safi A, Komzák M, et al. Platelet-rich plasma in patients with tibiofemoral cartilage degeneration. Arch Orthop Trauma Surg 2013;133(9):1295–301.

78. Civinini R, Nistri L, Martini C, et al. Growth factors in the treatment of early osteoarthritis. Clin Cases Miner Bone Metab 2013;10(1):26–9.

79. Carballo CB, Nakagawa Y, Sekiya I, et al. Basic science of articular cartilage. Clin Sports Med 2017;36(3):413–25.

80. Braun HJ, Kim HJ, Chu CR, et al. The effect of platelet-rich plasma formulations and blood products on human synoviocytes: implications for intra-articular injury and therapy. Am J Sports Med 2014;42(5):1204–10.

81. Bergeson AG, Tashjian RZ, Greis PE, et al. Effects of platelet-rich fibrin matrix on repair integrity of at-risk rotator cuff tears. Am J Sports Med 2012;40(2):286–93.

82. Castricini R, Longo UG, De Benedetto M, et al. Platelet-rich plasma augmentation for arthroscopic rotator cuff repair: a randomized controlled trial. Am J Sports Med 2011;39(2):258–65.

83. D'Ambrosi R, Palumbo F, Paronzini A, et al. Platelet-rich plasma supplementation in arthroscopic repair of full-thickness rotator cuff tears: a randomized clinical trial. Musculoskelet Surg 2016;100(S1):25–32.

84. Ebert JR, Wang A, Smith A, et al. A midterm evaluation of postoperative platelet-rich plasma injections on arthroscopic supraspinatus repair: a randomized controlled trial. Am J Sports Med 2017;45(13):2965–74.

85. Gumina S, Campagna V, Ferrazza G, et al. Use of platelet-leukocyte membrane in arthroscopic repair of large rotator cuff tears: a prospective randomized study. J Bone Joint Surg Am 2012;94(15):1345–52.

86. Holtby R, Christakis M, Maman E, et al. Impact of platelet-rich plasma on arthroscopic repair of small- to medium-sized rotator cuff tears: a randomized controlled trial. Orthop J Sports Med 2016;4(9). 232596711666559.

87. Jo CH, Shin JS, Shin WH, et al. Platelet-rich plasma for arthroscopic repair of medium to large rotator cuff tears: a randomized controlled trial. Am J Sports Med 2015;43(9):2102–10.

88. Malavolta EA, Gracitelli MEC, Ferreira Neto AA, et al. Platelet-rich plasma in rotator cuff repair: a prospective randomized study. Am J Sports Med 2014; 42(10):2446–54.

89. Randelli P, Arrigoni P, Ragone V, et al. Platelet rich plasma in arthroscopic rotator cuff repair: a prospective RCT study, 2-year follow-up. J Shoulder Elbow Surg 2011;20(4):518–28.

90. Rodeo SA, Delos D, Williams RJ, et al. The effect of platelet-rich fibrin matrix on rotator cuff tendon healing: a prospective, randomized clinical study. Am J Sports Med 2012;40(6):1234–41.

91. Weber SC, Kauffman JI, Parise C, et al. Platelet-rich fibrin matrix in the management of arthroscopic repair of the rotator cuff: a prospective, randomized, double-blinded study. Am J Sports Med 2013;41(2):263–70.

92. Zumstein MA, Rumian A, Thélu CÉ, et al. SECEC Research Grant 2008 II: Use of platelet- and leucocyte-rich fibrin (L-PRF) does not affect late rotator cuff tendon healing: a prospective randomized controlled study. J Shoulder Elbow Surg 2016;25(1):2–11.

93. Barber FA. Triple-loaded single-row versus suture-bridge double-row rotator cuff tendon repair with platelet-rich plasma fibrin membrane: a randomized controlled trial. Arthroscopy 2016;32(5):753–61.

94. Pandey V, Bandi A, Madi S, et al. Does application of moderately concentrated platelet-rich plasma improve clinical and structural outcome after arthroscopic repair of medium-sized to large rotator cuff tear? A randomized controlled trial. J Shoulder Elbow Surg 2016;25(8):1312–22.

95. Flury M, Rickenbacher D, Schwyzer H-K, et al. Does pure platelet-rich plasma affect postoperative clinical outcomes after arthroscopic rotator cuff repair? A randomized controlled trial. Am J Sports Med 2016;44(8):2136–46.

96. Cai Y, Zhang C, Lin X. Efficacy of platelet-rich plasma in arthroscopic repair of full-thickness rotator cuff tears: a meta-analysis. J Shoulder Elbow Surg 2015; 24(12):1852–9.

97. Saltzman BM, Jain A, Campbell KA, et al. Does the use of platelet-rich plasma at the time of surgery improve clinical outcomes in arthroscopic rotator cuff repair when compared with control cohorts? A systematic review of meta-analyses. Arthroscopy 2016;32(5):906–18.

98. Filardo G, Di Matteo B, Kon E, et al. Platelet-rich plasma in tendon-related disorders: results and indications. Knee Surg Sports Traumatol Arthrosc 2018; 26(7):1984–99.

99. Vavken P, Sadoghi P, Palmer M, et al. Platelet-rich plasma reduces retear rates after arthroscopic repair of small- and medium-sized rotator cuff tears but is not cost-effective. Am J Sports Med 2015;43(12):3071–6.

100. Smith KM, Le A, Costouros J, et al. Biologics for rotator cuff repair: a critical analysis review. JBJS Rev, in press.

101. Allahverdi A, Sharifi D, Takhtfooladi MA, et al. Evaluation of low-level laser therapy, platelet-rich plasma, and their combination on the healing of Achilles tendon in rabbits. Lasers Med Sci 2015;30(4):1305–13.

102. Chen L, Dong SW, Liu JP, et al. Synergy of tendon stem cells and platelet-rich plasma in tendon healing. J Orthop Res 2012;30(6):991–7.

103. Kaux JF, Drion PV, Colige A, et al. Effects of platelet-rich plasma (PRP) on the healing of Achilles tendons of rats. Wound Repair Regen 2012;20(5):748–56.

104. Kim HJ, Nam HW, Hur CY, et al. The effect of platelet rich plasma from bone marrow aspirate with added bone morphogenetic protein-2 on the Achilles tendon-bone junction in rabbits. Clin Orthop Surg 2011;3(4):325–31.

105. Lyras DN, Kazakos K, Georgiadis G, et al. Does a single application of PRP alter the expression of IGF-I in the early phase of tendon healing? J Foot Ankle Surg 2011;50(3):276–82.

106. Lyras DN, Kazakos K, Tryfonidis M, et al. Temporal and spatial expression of TGF-beta1 in an Achilles tendon section model after application of platelet-rich plasma. Foot Ankle Surg 2010;16(3):137–41.

107. Yuksel S, Gulec MA, Gultekin MZ, et al. Comparison of the early period effects of bone marrow-derived mesenchymal stem cells and platelet-rich plasma on the Achilles tendon ruptures in rats. Connect Tissue Res 2016;57(5):360–73.

108. Sadoghi P, Rosso C, Valderrabano V, et al. The role of platelets in the treatment of Achilles tendon injuries. J Orthop Res 2013;31(1):111–8.

109. Aspenberg P. Platelet concentrates and Achilles tendon healing. J Orthop Res 2013;31(9):1500.

110. Andersson T, Eliasson P, Hammerman M, et al. Low-level mechanical stimulation is sufficient to improve tendon healing in rats. J Appl Physiol 1985 2012;113(9): 1398–402.

111. Virchenko O, Aspenberg P. How can one platelet injection after tendon injury lead to a stronger tendon after 4 weeks? Interplay between early regeneration and mechanical stimulation. Acta Orthop 2006;77(5):806–12.

112. Schepull T, Kvist J, Norrman H, et al. Autologous platelets have no effect on the healing of human Achilles tendon ruptures: a randomized single-blind study. Am J Sports Med 2011;39(1):38–47.

113. De Carli A, Lanzetti RM, Ciompi A, et al. Can platelet-rich plasma have a role in Achilles tendon surgical repair? Knee Surg Sports Traumatol Arthrosc 2016; 24(7):2231–7.

114. Zou J, Mo X, Shi Z, et al. A prospective study of platelet-rich plasma as biological augmentation for acute Achilles tendon rupture repair. Biomed Res Int 2016; 2016:1–8.

115. Di Matteo B, Loibl M, Andriolo L, et al. Biologic agents for anterior cruciate ligament healing: a systematic review. World J Orthop 2016;7(9):592–603.

116. Orrego M, Larrain C, Rosales J, et al. Effects of platelet concentrate and a bone plug on the healing of hamstring tendons in a bone tunnel. Arthroscopy 2008; 24(12):1373–80.

117. Radice F, Yánez R, Gutiérrez V, et al. Comparison of magnetic resonance imaging findings in anterior cruciate ligament grafts with and without autologous platelet-derived growth factors. Arthroscopy 2010;26(1):50–7.

118. Seijas R, Ares O, Catala J, et al. Magnetic resonance imaging evaluation of patellar tendon graft remodelling after anterior cruciate ligament reconstruction with or without platelet-rich plasma. J Orthop Surg (Hong Kong) 2013;21(1): 10–4.

119. Sánchez M, Anitua E, Azofra J, et al. Ligamentization of tendon grafts treated with an endogenous preparation rich in growth factors: gross morphology and histology. Arthroscopy 2010;26(4):470–80.

120. Nin JRV, Gasque GM, Azcárate AV, et al. Has platelet-rich plasma any role in anterior cruciate ligament allograft healing? Arthroscopy 2009;25(11):1206–13.

121. Vogrin M, Rupreht M, Dinevski D, et al. Effects of a platelet gel on early graft revascularization after anterior cruciate ligament reconstruction: a prospective, randomized, double-blind, clinical trial. Eur Surg Res 2010;45(2):77–85.

122. Andriolo L, Di Matteo B, Kon E, et al. PRP augmentation for ACL reconstruction. Biomed Res Int 2015;2015:1–15.

123. Mirzatolooei F, Alamdari MT, Khalkhali HR. The impact of platelet-rich plasma on the prevention of tunnel widening in anterior cruciate ligament reconstruction using quadrupled autologous hamstring tendon. Bone Joint J 2013;95-B(1):65–9.

124. Figueroa D, Melean P, Calvo R, et al. Magnetic resonance imaging evaluation of the integration and maturation of semitendinosus-gracilis graft in anterior cruciate ligament reconstruction using autologous platelet concentrate. Arthroscopy 2010;26(10):1318–25.

125. Ventura A, Terzaghi C, Borgo E, et al. Use of growth factors in ACL surgery: preliminary study. J Orthop Traumatol 2005;6(2):76–9.

126. de Almeida AM, Demange MK, Sobrado MF, et al. Patellar tendon healing with platelet-rich plasma: a prospective randomized controlled trial. Am J Sports Med 2012;40(6):1282–8.

127. Seijas R, Cuscó X, Sallent A, et al. Pain in donor site after BTB-ACL reconstruction with PRGF: a randomized trial. Arch Orthop Trauma Surg 2016;136(6): 829–35.

128. Cervellin M, de Girolamo L, Bait C, et al. Autologous platelet-rich plasma gel to reduce donor-site morbidity after patellar tendon graft harvesting for anterior cruciate ligament reconstruction: a randomized, controlled clinical study. Knee Surg Sports Traumatol Arthrosc 2012;20(1):114–20.

129. Rowden A, Dominici P, D'Orazio J, et al. Double-blind, randomized, placebo-controlled study evaluating the use of Platelet-rich Plasma Therapy (PRP) for acute ankle sprains in the emergency department. J Emerg Med 2015;49(4): 546–51.

130. Laver L, Carmont MR, McConkey MO, et al. Plasma rich in growth factors (PRGF) as a treatment for high ankle sprain in elite athletes: a randomized control trial. Knee Surg Sports Traumatol Arthrosc 2015;23(11):3383–92.

131. A Hamid MS, Mohamed Ali MR, Yusof A, et al. Platelet-rich plasma injections for the treatment of hamstring injuries: a randomized controlled trial. Am J Sports Med 2014;42(10):2410–8.

132. Reurink G, Goudswaard GJ, Moen MH, et al. Platelet-rich plasma injections in acute muscle injury. N Engl J Med 2014;370(26):2546–7.

133. Li H, Usas A, Poddar M, et al. Platelet-rich plasma promotes the proliferation of human muscle derived progenitor cells and maintains their stemness. PLoS One 2013;8(6):e64923.

134. Artaza JN, Bhasin S, Magee TR, et al. Myostatin inhibits myogenesis and promotes adipogenesis in C3H 10T(1/2) mesenchymal multipotent cells. Endocrinology 2005;146(8):3547–57.

135. Burks TN, Cohn RD. Role of TGF-β signaling in inherited and acquired myopathies. Skelet Muscle 2011;1(1):19.

136. Miroshnychenko O, Chang W, Dragoo JL. The use of platelet-rich and platelet-poor plasma to enhance differentiation of skeletal myoblasts: implications for the use of autologous blood products for muscle regeneration. Am J Sports Med 2017;45(4):945–53.

137. Marcazzan S, Taschieri S, Weinstein RL, et al. Efficacy of platelet concentrates in bone healing: a systematic review on animal studies—Part B: large-size animal models. Platelets 2018;29(4):338–46.

138. Roffi A, Di Matteo B, Krishnakumar GS, et al. Platelet-rich plasma for the treatment of bone defects: from pre-clinical rational to evidence in the clinical practice. A systematic review. Int Orthop 2017;41(2):221–37.

139. Cho K, Kim JM, Kim MH, et al. Scintigraphic evaluation of osseointegrative response around calcium phosphate-coated titanium implants in tibia bone: effect of platelet-rich plasma on bone healing in dogs. Eur Surg Res 2013;51(3–4): 138–45.

140. Archundia TR, Soriano JC, Corona JN. Utility of platelet-rich plasma and growth factors bone in the bone defects. Regional Hospital Lic. Adolfo Lopez Mateos, ISSSTE. Acta Ortop Mex 2007;21(5):256–60 [in Spanish].

141. Batista MA, Leivas TP, Rodrigues CJ, et al. Comparison between the effects of platelet-rich plasma and bone marrow concentrate on defect consolidation in the rabbit tibia. Clinics (Sao Paulo) 2011;66(10):1787–92.

142. Dulgeroglu TC, Metineren H. Evaluation of the effect of platelet-rich fibrin on long bone healing: an experimental rat model. Orthopedics 2017;40(3):e479–84.

143. Gianakos A, Zambrana L, Savage-Elliott I, et al. Platelet-rich plasma in the animal long-bone model: an analysis of basic science evidence. Orthopedics 2015;38(12):e1079–90.
144. Guzel Y, Karalezli N, Bilge O, et al. The biomechanical and histological effects of platelet-rich plasma on fracture healing. Knee Surg Sports Traumatol Arthrosc 2015;23(5):1378–83.
145. Simman R, Hoffmann A, Bohinc RJ, et al. Role of platelet-rich plasma in acceleration of bone fracture healing. Ann Plast Surg 2008;61(3):337–44.
146. Zhang N, Wu YP, Qian SJ, et al. Research progress in the mechanism of effect of PRP in bone deficiency healing. ScientificWorldJournal 2013;2013:134582.
147. Cheng X, Lei D, Mao T, et al. Repair of critical bone defects with injectable platelet rich plasma/bone marrow-derived stromal cells composite: experimental study in rabbits. Ulus Travma Acil Cerrahi Derg 2008;14(2):87–95.
148. Kanthan SR, Kavitha G, Addi S, et al. Platelet-rich plasma (PRP) enhances bone healing in non-united critical-sized defects: a preliminary study involving rabbit models. Injury 2011;42(8):782–9.
149. Sarkar MR, Augat P, Shefelbine SJ, et al. Bone formation in a long bone defect model using a platelet-rich plasma-loaded collagen scaffold. Biomaterials 2006; 27(9):1817–23.
150. Calori GM, Tagliabue L, Gala L, et al. Application of rhBMP-7 and platelet-rich plasma in the treatment of long bone non-unions: a prospective randomised clinical study on 120 patients. Injury 2008;39(12):1391–402.

Amniotic-Derived Treatments and Formulations

Robert A. Duerr, MD[a],*, Jakob Ackermann, MD[b],
Andreas H. Gomoll, MD[c]

KEYWORDS

- Amniotic membrane • Amniotic fluid • Allograft • Sports medicine injury
- Tissue regeneration

KEY POINTS

- Amniotic-derived products have been used for decades in various medical subspecialties and are safe for allograft transplantation.
- These products show promising preclinical and early clinical results in the treatment of tendon/ligament injuries, cartilage defects, and osteoarthritis.
- The therapeutic benefits of amniotic-derived products are likely due to intrinsic properties, such as their structure as an extracellular matrix and concentration of growth factors, as well as anti-inflammatory, antifibrotic, and antimicrobial molecules.
- High-quality clinical trials are needed to elucidate the specific applications and benefits of these individual products for orthopedic sports medicine indications.

INTRODUCTION

Orthobiologics are increasingly used by orthopedic surgeons to enhance healing of injured tissues, such as bone, muscle, tendon, ligament, and articular cartilage. These products are derived from substances that are naturally occurring in the human body and can be composed of growth factors (eg, bone morphogenic proteins), cells (eg, mesenchymal stem cells [MSCs]), or a combination thereof (eg, platelet rich plasma and amniotic-derived products). MSCs, or multipotent progenitor cells, have been an important area of investigation due to their ability to differentiate into various cell

Disclosures: A.H. Gomoll receives research support, consulting fees, and royalties from Organogenesis Inc, Canton, MA. R.A. Duerr and J. Ackermann have no commercial or financial disclosures.
[a] Department of Orthopedic surgery, Jameson Crane Sports Medicine Institute, Ohio State University, 2835 Fred Taylor Drive, Columbus, OH 43202, USA; [b] Department of Orthopedic Surgery, Brigham & Women's Hospital, 75 Francis Street, Boston, MA 02115, USA; [c] Department of Orthopedic surgery, Hospital for Special Surgery, Weill-Cornell Medical School, 535 East 70th Street, New York, NY 10021, USA
* Corresponding author.
E-mail address: robbie.duerr@gmail.com

Clin Sports Med 38 (2019) 45–59
https://doi.org/10.1016/j.csm.2018.08.002
0278-5919/19/© 2018 Elsevier Inc. All rights reserved.

sportsmed.theclinics.com

types in mesenchymal tissues and to secrete a large number of bioactive macromolecules important in the tissue regenerative process.[1]

MSCs are a subtype of adult stem cells that are found throughout the body and have been isolated from human bone marrow, adipose, muscle, and synovial tissue.[1-3] Although adult-derived MSCs have demonstrated promising clinical applications, several limitations exist. The number of MSCs in marrow tissues is limited, and after skeletal maturity this supply becomes even less robust.[4] Donor site morbidity from autologous harvest, primarily pain at the donor site, can be a significant complication.[5] In addition, the Food and Drug Administration (FDA) allows for only minimal manipulation of autologous MSCs. For these reasons, researchers are continually investigating alternative sources of MSCs, including placental-derived tissues, such as the amniotic membrane (AM), amniotic fluid (AF), umbilical cord, and umbilical cord blood.[6] For the purposes of this review, the authors focus on products derived from the AM and fluid.

Amniotic tissues have been used for more than 100 years in the treatment of burn wounds, and other medical subspecialties, although it has only been recently that these tissues have been investigated for orthopedic applications.[7] The AM has been shown to be a rich source of MSCs, which show a greater differentiation plasticity and higher proliferative potential.[8] In addition to the stem cells present in these tissues, the AM is a metabolically active tissue that has demonstrated anti-inflammatory, antimicrobial, antifibrotic, and epithelialization-promoting features that make it uniquely suited for several clinical applications.[8]

ANATOMY AND FUNCTIONS OF THE AMNIOTIC MEMBRANE

The AM is composed of 3 distinct layers: epithelium, basement membrane, and outer mesenchymal layer. The innermost epithelial layer is composed of a single layer of flat cuboidal cells with the apical surface having a brush border with many microvilli active in secretory and cellular transport functions.[9] These amniotic epithelial cells (AECs) are derived from the developing epiblast and therefore share some of the features of pluripotent embryonic stem cells and have the ability to differentiate into all 3 germ layers (ectoderm, mesoderm, and endoderm). The underlying basement membrane is one of the thickest basement membranes in human tissue and is composed of laminins, type IV and VII collagen, and fibronectin. The basement membrane separates the epithelium from the outer mesenchyme, which consists of 3 distinct layers: compact, fibroblast, and intermediate or spongy layer. The compact stromal layer is the strongest of the AM and contains bundles of collagen, elastic fibers, hyaluronic acid, and proteoglycans. A network of fibroblasts and few macrophages compose the fibroblast layer, which produces type I and III collagens that form parallel bundles to give structural integrity to the AM. Also, type V and VI collagens create crosslinks between the basement membrane and stromal layers. The outer spongy layer contains several glycoproteins and proteoglycans along with a nonfibrillar network of type III collagen that loosely connects with the chorionic mesoderm.[10]

The structural integrity of the AM provides an extracellular matrix that can serve as a scaffold for cellular migration and proliferation to enhance wound healing and epithelialization.[10,11] Several growth factors important for epithelialization are produced by the amniotic mesenchymal and epithelial cells. The antifibrotic properties of the AM are thought to be due primarily to the secretion of tissue inhibitors of metalloproteinases (MMPs) and the downregulation of transforming growth factor-beta (TGF-β), which normally activates fibroblasts.[11]

Other factors produced by the AM have substantial anti-inflammatory effects, such as a unique heavy chain–hyaluronic acid, which has been shown to inhibit the complement cascade and influence the activation of macrophages.[12] The AM also suppresses proinflammatory cytokines interleukin-1-alpha (IL-1α), IL-1β, and TGF-β. The production of natural MMP inhibitors by the AM may further reduce inflammation.[13]

The AM has antimicrobial properties as a structural barrier and through the production of several antimicrobial molecules.[14] It is also an immunoprivileged tissue, in that AECs do not express major histocompatibility antigens (HLA classes A, B, DR). This property is directly related to the reduced risk of rejection or immune reaction when used as an allograft.[15]

AMNIOTIC-DERIVED PRODUCTS

In the United States, the market for amniotic-derived products is rapidly expanding, and each company's processing, storage, and delivery methods are variable. These products are available as a sheet or injectable suspension. Sheets are composed of one or more layers of the placental membrane: amnion, amnion and chorion, double layer amnion, or umbilical cord.[16] Injectable products, or amnion suspension allografts (ASAs), are typically composed of micronized amnion and/or chorion in a suspension of AF.[7,16]

The commercially available amniotic-derived products in the United States are classified as Human Cells, Tissues, and Cellular and Tissue-Based Products and are subject to regulation by the FDA under section 361 of the Public Health Service Act. These products must satisfy 4 criteria: minimal manipulation, homologous use, not combined with drugs or devices, and not reliant on cell metabolic activity as a primary function.[17] Some products may not meet these criteria and be considered a biologic drug under section 351, requiring a Biologics License Application and Investigational New Drug application, which is much more time consuming and costly.[7]

Amniotic-derived products are obtained from placenta shortly after caesarean delivery in consenting adults who have undergone serologic screening for communicable diseases, including human immunodeficiency virus, hepatitis B and C, human T-cell lymphotropic virus, and syphilis.[18] The placentas are aseptically collected and typically washed with antibiotic-containing solution to cover gram-positive and gram-negative bacteria as well as fungi (penicillin, streptomycin, neomycin, and amphotericin B).[18] The AM can be separated from the chorion by blunt dissection and is preserved by means of cryopreservation, dehydration, or fresh cold storage depending on each company's protocol.[16,18]

The cryopreservation process involves washing of the AM and storage at −80°C in a cryoprotectant media such as glycerol or dimethylsulfoxide.[19] With cryopreservation, the native cells are thought to be preserved, although studies have demonstrated variable cell viability with cryopreservation techniques. Dehydration can be accomplished through several techniques to remove water content, such as lyophilization (freeze drying), desiccation, or dry heating. The various processing methods can decrease mechanical strength and reduce the amount of total protein and growth factors in the AM.[19,20] However, the extracellular matrix components and structural integrity of the basement membrane are maintained, which may be the most important for influencing cell adhesion and reducing scar formation.[19,20]

CLINICAL APPLICATIONS IN SPORTS MEDICINE

The safety and efficacy of amniotic tissues have been demonstrated through years of use in other medical subspecialties, although the existing literature describing their use in orthopedic sports medicine is limited. A recent systematic review identified 29 animal studies and 6 human studies reporting the use of placenta-derived cells and placental tissue allografts for orthopedic sports medicine indications.[17] Because this review focuses on the use of amniotic-derived products, studies investigating the use of umbilical cord blood MSCs were excluded, and several additional studies were identified, resulting in 20 animal studies (**Table 1**) and 7 human studies (**Table 2**).

ANIMAL MODELS
Articular Cartilage Injury

The use of amniotic-derived products for the treatment of articular cartilage injuries has demonstrated promising results. Nogami and colleagues[21] used human amniotic membrane mesenchymal stem cells (hAM-MSCs) in culture with a polylactic-*co*-gly-colic acid (PLGA) scaffold to treat chondral defects created in the trochlea of rats, resulting in regenerative tissue with strong staining for type II collagen, and significantly better cartilage scores than the control groups at 24 weeks. In a similar rat model, using a collagen scaffold in combination with hAM-MSCs implanted into femoral condyle defects, Wei and colleagues[22] demonstrated filling of the defects with hyaline-like cartilage. Garcia and colleagues[23] compared the results of fresh sheep AM, cryopreserved sheep AM, and cryopreserved sheep AM combined with bone marrow–derived MSCs. At 2 months, all groups demonstrated improved International Cartilage Repair Society and O'Driscoll scores versus controls, although this did not reach statistical significance. In another sheep model, Tabet and colleagues[24] demonstrated filling of full-thickness defects with hyaline-like cartilage using human AM combined with demineralize bone matrix. Jin and colleagues[25] evaluated the feasibility of hAM as a carrier of rabbit chondrocytes and demonstrated cell proliferation and maintenance with expression of type II collagen on hAM. The hAM seeded with rabbit chondrocytes was then implanted into femoral condyle defects in rabbits and at 8 weeks had regenerated hyaline-like cartilage.[25]

Knee Osteoarthritis

Willett and colleagues[26] injected micronized dehydrated human amniotic and chorionic membrane (mdHACM) into the knees of rats 24 hours after the rats underwent surgical transection of the medial meniscus to induce osteoarthritis. Treatment reduced the number and severity of chondral lesions and helped maintain higher proteoglycan content versus controls injected with saline, concluding that treatment showed a chondroprotective effect against the development of osteoarthritis. Kim and colleagues[27] used injectable human placental extract (HPE) in the knees of rats treated with monoiodoacetate (MIA) to induce osteoarthritis. HPE significantly reduced the development of a deformity in the knees and suppressed the histologic changes in MIA-induced osteoarthritis. They thought this chondroprotective effect may be due to suppression of matrix MMP-2 and MMP-9.

Tendon and Ligament Injury

The use of amniotic-derived products for the treatment of Achilles tendon injuries in animal models has demonstrated variable results. Coban and colleagues[28] found no significant differences in the histopathology or mechanical strength of surgically repaired rat Achilles tendons augmented with human AF injection or hAM wrap versus tendon repair alone at 3 weeks and concluded that treatment showed no improvement in rat tendon healing in the early phase.

Table 1
Summary of animal studies using amniotic-derived products for orthopedic sports medicine indications

Study (Year)	Indication	Animal Model	Amniotic Product	Treatment	Results
Nogami et al,[21] 2016	Articular cartilage injury	Rat	ECM from human AM-MSCs	Defect in trochlear groove 1. Control 2. PLGA alone 3. PLGA + ECM	PLGA + ECM resulted in hyaline cartilage Cartilage score significantly improved at 24 wk vs controls
Garcia et al,[23] 2015	Articular cartilage injury	Sheep	Sheep AM	Defect in WB femoral condyle 1. Control 2. Fresh AM 3. Cryopreserved AM + BM-MSCs 4. Cryopreserved AM	At 2 mo, all groups demonstrated improved ICRS and O'Driscoll scores vs controls No differences between experimental groups
Tabet et al,[24] 2015	Articular cartilage injury	Sheep	Human AM + DBX	Defects in femoral condyle and trochlea filled with 1. Control 2. Human AM + DBX	Experimental group demonstrated fill of defects with stromal matrix similar to hyaline cartilage
Wei et al,[22] 2009	Articular cartilage injury	Rat	Human amniotic MSCs	Defect in femoral condyle treated with human amniotic MSCs in collagen scaffold + BMP-2	Demonstrated filling of defects with hyaline-like cartilage
Jin et al,[25] 2007	Articular cartilage injury	Rabbit	Fresh human AM; denuded human AM	Rabbit chondrocytes seeded on 1. Fresh human AM 2. Basement side of denuded AM 3. Stromal side of denuded AM	Chondrocytes preferentially grew and expressed type II collagen on stromal side of denuded AM Regenerated hyaline cartilage in femoral condyle defects
Willett et al,[26] 2014	Knee osteoarthritis	Rat	mdHACM	Rats underwent transection of medial meniscus to induce OA 24 h postoperatively injected with 1. mdHACM 2. Saline	Treatment reduced the number and severity of chondral lesions Helped maintain higher proteoglycan content

(continued on next page)

Table 1
(continued)

Study (Year)	Indication	Animal Model	Amniotic Product	Treatment	Results
Kim et al,[27] 2010	Knee osteoarthritis	Rat	Human placenta extract	MIA injection induced OA model in rats after 14 d received daily injection for 14 d 1. Saline 2. Differing doses of HPE	Significantly reduced deformity and histologic changes with HPE
Kueckelhaus et al,[33] 2014	Achilles tendon	Rat	Human ACCS	Achilles transected, ends injected then repaired 1. Saline 2. ACCS in carboxymethyl cellulose	Group 2 showed significantly higher strength at 2, 4, and 6 wk vs controls and higher crosslink density At 8 wk, controls showed significantly higher strength
Philip et al,[32] 2013	Achilles tendon	Rat	Human AMPCs; ACCS	Achilles transected, ends injected then repaired 1. Saline 2. ACCS 3. AMPCs	At 4 wk, significantly improved mechanical strength in group 3 vs 2 and controls
Barboni et al,[30] 2012	Achilles tendon	Sheep	Sheep AECs	Achilles defect created and treated with 1. Sheep AECs 2. Control	AEC-treated tendons demonstrated improved mechanical properties, ECM remodeling, and collagen maturation vs controls
Muttini et al,[29] 2010	Achilles tendon	Sheep	Sheep AECs	Bilateral Achilles defects created with collagenase injections 1. AECs injected at 15 d 2. No injection contralateral leg	AEC treated tendons showed active proliferation of reparative cells and organization of neo-collagen at 30 d
Coban et al,[28] 2009	Achilles tendon	Rat	Human AF; Fresh AM	Steroid induced tendinosis then cut and repaired with 1. Suture repair only 2. Suture + AF injection 3. Suture + AF + AM wrap	At 3 wk, no difference in histopathology or mechanical strength
Özbölük et al,[36] 2010	Flexor tendon	Rabbit	Human AM	Flexor tendon transected 1. Repair alone 2. Repair + AM wrap 3. Repair + periosteal autograft wrap	Group 3 biomechanically strongest at 2 and 6 wk Group 2 stronger at wk 2, but not 6 vs controls Less adhesions in groups 2 and 3 vs controls at 6 wk

Study	Animal	Injury	Material	Procedure/Groups	Results
Özgenel et al,[34] 2004	Chicken	Flexor tendon	Human fresh AM + HA	50% partial tenotomy: 1. Repair alone 2. Repair + AM wrap 3. Repair + HA injection 4. Repair + AM wrap + HA injection	Group 4 demonstrated least amount of adhesion and best motion; Group 2 and 3 less adhesion and better motion than controls; No significant differences in strength
Demirkan et al,[37] 2002	Chicken	Flexor tendon	Human fresh AM	Flexor tendon transected: 1. Repair tendon alone 2. Repair tendon + sheath 3. Repair tendon + sheath + AM wrap around tendon repair	Group 3 demonstrated reduced adhesion formation and no differences in strength of repairs
Özgenel et al,[35] 2001	Rabbit	Flexor tendon	Human AF	Flexor tendon transected and repaired with: 1. Sheath excised 2. Sheath excised + AF applied 3. Sheath repaired 4. Sheath repaired + AF applied	Group 4 demonstrated best healing and least adhesion; Significantly better load to failure in groups treated with AF
Muttini et al,[39] 2015	Horse	Acute/chronic tendon lesion	Sheep AECs	Acute/chronic flexor tendinopathy injected with cultured sheep AECs	At 180 d, histology showed complete restoration of normal tendon architecture
Muttini et al,[38] 2013	Horse	Acute/chronic tendon lesion	Sheep AECs	Acute or chronic flexor tendon lesions confirmed by US: 1. Control 2. Injection of sheep AECs	Treatment group demonstrated integration of sheep AECs and production of type 1 collagen; Increased echogenicity, cross-sectional area, and fiber alignment by 3 mo after injection
Lange-Consiglio et al,[40] 2013	Horse	Tendon and/or ligament injury	Horse AM-MSCs	Tendon or ligament injury randomized to injection with: 1. Horse AM-MSCs 2. BM-MSCs	AM-MSCs resulted in faster average return to activity and decreased reinjury rates for 2 y vs BM-MSCs
Lange-Consiglio et al,[41] 2013	Horse	Tendon and/or ligament injury	Horse amniotic MSC–conditioned medium	Tendon or ligament injury injected with horse MSC–conditioned medium vs controls	Treatment significantly reduced reinjury rate vs controls

Abbreviations: BM, bone marrow; BMP, bone morphogenic protein; DBX, demineralized bone matrix; ECM, extracellular matrix; HA, hyaluronic acid; ICRS, International Cartilage Repair Society; OA, osteoarthritis; US, ultrasound; WB, weight bearing.

Table 2
Summary of human studies using amniotic derived products for orthopedic sports medicine indications

Study (Year)	Indication	Study Design	Amniotic Product	n	Treatment	Study Time Points	Outcome Measures	Safety	Results
Vines et al,[48] 2016	Knee OA	Prospective open-label case series	Cryopreserved micronized AM and AF (Renu)	6	Symptomatic OA, single intra-articular injection of 2 mL Renu + 2 mL saline	1 and 2 wk 3, 6, and 12 mo	Blood/serum analysis IKDC, KOOS, SANE scores	2 patients with transient pain increase	General trend toward improvement in all PROMs Significant increase in IgG and IgE, though still within normal limits
Gellhorn & Han,[47] 2017	Degenerative arthritis or tendinopathy	Retrospective case series	dHACM (Amniofix)	40	US-guided injection of 40 mg Amniofix in 1 mL saline	1, 2, and 3 mo	VAS, PSFS	Localized pain for mean 2.25 d, no serious adverse events	Significant improvement in patient's pain and function at 1, 2, and 3 mo
Werber,[44] 2015	Plantar fasciitis, Achilles tendinosis	Prospective open-label case series	Cryopreserved micronized AM and AF (SportFlow)	44	US-guided injection of 0.5 mL SportFlow + 0.5 mL 1% Lidocaine in plantar fasciitis; 1 mL SportFlow + 1 mL 1% lidocaine in Achilles tendinosis	2, 4, 6, 8, 10, and 12 wk	VAS	No treatment-related adverse events reported	VAS pain scores significantly improved in all patients by 4 wk, and improvements were maintained up to 12 wk

Study	Condition	Product	Study Design	N	Methods	Follow-up	Outcome Measures	Adverse Events	Results
Hanselman et al,[42] 2015	Plantar fasciitis	Cryopreserved micronized AM (ClarixFlo)	Prospective, randomized, controlled, double-blind pilot study	23	Patients randomized to injection with ClarixFlo vs corticosteroid and option for repeat injection at 6 wk	6, 12, and 18 wk	FHSQ, VAS, verbal % improvement	No adverse events reported	No significant differences in patients receiving only 1 injection; There was significant improvement in FHSQ foot pain score in 2 injection ClarixFlo group vs steroid; Verbal % improvement at 12 wk was greater in steroid group vs ClarixFlo
Zelen et al,[43] 2013	Plantar fasciitis	mdHACM (Amniofix injectable)	Prospective, randomized, controlled, single-blind study	45	Patients randomized to injection of 0.5% Marcaine and (1) saline, (2) 0.5 mL mdHACM, (3) 1.25 mL mdHACM	8 wk	AOFAS, Wong-Baker Faces pain rating scale, SF-36	No adverse events reported	All outcome measures significantly improved in both treatment groups vs no improvement in saline group
Lullove,[45] 2015	Foot and ankle tendonitis	Flowable placental tissue matrix allograft (PX50)	Retrospective case series	10	Patients with acute or chronic tendon injury received injection with 1 mL 0.5% bupivacaine + 0.5 mL PX50	6 wk	VAS	No adverse events reported	All patients' pain resolved to VAS of 0 by 5 wk
Warner & Lasyone,[46] 2014	Foot/ankle surgery	Cryopreserved AM and umbilical cord (Clarix Cord 1k)	Retrospective case series	14	Patients undergoing revision or complex foot and ankle surgery involving tendon or nerve had Clarix Cord applied intraoperatively	Range 4-32 wk	AOFAS, NRS	No adverse events reported	Postoperative AOFAS and NRS scores were significantly improved at final follow-up vs preoperative scores

Abbreviations: FHSQ, Foot Health Status Questionnaire; IgE, immunoglobulin E; IgG, immunoglobulin G; IKDC, International Knee Documentation Committee; KOOS, Knee Injury and Osteoarthritis Outcome Score; mdHACM, micronized dehydrated human amniotic/chorionic membrane; OA, osteoarthritis; PROMs, patient reported outcome measures; PSFS, Patient-Specific Functional Scale; SANE, single assessment numeric evaluation; SF-36, 36-item Short Form health survey; US, ultrasound.

Two similar studies using AECs to treat Achilles tendon defects in a sheep model demonstrated favorable results. The AEC-treated tendons demonstrated active proliferation of reparative cells and organization of neo-collagen, improved mechanical properties, ECM remodeling, and collagen maturation in treatment group versus controls.[29,30]

Amnion-derived cellular cytokine solution (ACCS) is the supernatant of cultured amnion-derived multipotent progenitor cells (AMPCs) and contains physiologic levels of cytokines important to the healing process.[31] Philip and colleagues[32] performed surgical repair of transected rat Achilles tendons augmented with ACCS or AMPCs versus controls. They demonstrated significant improvements in mechanical properties in the AMPC group over controls, but not in the ACCS group. In a similar study, Kueckelhaus and colleagues[33] augmented surgical repair of transected rat Achilles tendons with ACCS in a carboxymethyl cellulose scaffold. They demonstrated significantly higher strength and crosslink density in the treatment group at 2, 4, and 6 weeks; however, at 8 weeks the control group demonstrated significantly higher strength. They concluded that the delivery of the ACCS in a slow release media likely improves its effects in the early phases of tendon healing.

Similar to the results in Achilles tendon injury models, the use of amniotic-derived products to augment flexor tendon repairs has been variable in improving repair strength, although AM used as a wrap for flexor tendon repair did demonstrate decreased adhesions and better motion in several studies.[34–37] Using injectable sheep AECs in the treatment of acute and chronic tendon injuries and horses, Muttini and colleagues[38,39] demonstrated integration of the sheep AECs and production of type 1 collagen with restoration of normal tendon architecture at 180 days. Lange-Consiglio and colleagues[40,41] reported 2 studies in horses with tendon or ligament injuries. In the first, they found the AM-MSC group had a faster average return to activity and decreased reinjury rate for 2 years of follow-up versus BM-MSCs.[40] In the second, they found injection with horse AM-MSC–conditioned medium also significantly reduced reinjury rates versus controls.[41]

HUMAN STUDIES

Of the 7 available (to date) human studies, 5 were for the treatment of foot and ankle conditions, one was a review of all patients from a single practice with degenerative arthritis or tendinopathy in various body areas, and one was a pilot study investigating the use of injectable micronized AM and AF for knee osteoarthritis. In the only randomized, controlled, double-blind study, Hanselman and colleagues[42] compared a cryopreserved micronized human AM (ClarixFlo; Amniox Medical Inc, Atlanta, GA, USA) to corticosteroid injections for plantar fasciitis in 23 patients. Patients also had the option of a repeat injection at their 6-week follow-up, and 3 patients from each group received a second injection. The investigators found no significant differences between groups when receiving only one injection. They did show a significant improvement in Foot Health Status Questionnaire pain score in the 2-injection ClarixFlo group versus corticosteroid at 18 weeks. Nonetheless, the corticosteroid group had significantly higher verbal percentage improvement at 12 weeks. They concluded that the injectable cryopreserved micronized AM may be safe and comparable to corticosteroid in the treatment of refractory plantar fasciitis.[42]

Zelen and colleagues[43] performed a randomized, controlled, single-blind feasibility study to treat chronic refractory plantar fasciitis. Forty-five patients were randomized to receive an injection of 2 mL of 0.5% Marcaine followed by either saline, 0.5 mL mdHACM (Amniofix injectable; Mimedx Group Inc, Marietta, GA, USA), or

1.25 mL mdHACM. At 8 weeks of follow-up, patients receiving mdHACM demonstrated significant improvements in all outcome measures at all study time points versus saline controls. There were no differences between the high and low doses of mdHACM, and no adverse events were reported over the study period.

Werber[44] performed a prospective, open-label case series using a cryopreserved micronized AM and AF (SportFlow; Amnio Technology, Phoenix, AZ, USA) injection to treat patients with plantar fasciitis and Achilles tendinosis who failed at least 6 months of prior treatment. Patients were followed for 12 weeks and had significant improvements in visual analog scale pain scores (VAS) by 4 weeks, which were maintained through the 12-week study period. Similar to Zelen and colleagues,[43] these early clinical results are promising, but the conclusions are limited due to the short-term follow-up.

Lullove[45] reported a retrospective case series of 10 patients who received injection with 0.5% bupivacaine + flowable placental tissue matrix allograft (PX50 BioRenew PTM Therapy; Skye Biologics Inc, El Segundo, CA, USA) for acute or chronic tendon injuries of the lower extremity. Patients were followed for 6 weeks and demonstrated complete resolution of pain by 5 weeks. Again, the conclusions of this report are limited due to small sample size, short-term follow-up, and lack of a control group.

Warner and Lasyone[46] reported a retrospective case series of patients undergoing revision or complex foot and ankle surgery with tendon and/or nerve interventions augmented with a cryopreserved human AM and umbilical cord matrix (Clarix Cord 1k Regenerative Matrix; Amniox Medical Inc, Atlanta, GA). Outcomes were assessed using the American Orthopedic Foot and Ankle Society (AOFAS) Ankle-Hindfoot Scale and pain numerical rating scale (NRS) scores. Fourteen patients were included in the review, and at a mean follow-up of 16 weeks (range: 4–32 weeks), they demonstrated significant improvements in postoperative AOFAS and NRS compared with preoperative scores.

Gellhorn and Han[47] performed a prospective case series of consecutive patients being treated for arthritis or tendinopathy with an ultrasound-guided injection of dHACM (Amniofix; Mimedx). Forty patients were included in the final analysis, including 8 knee, 2 tibiotalar, 2 subtalar, 3 glenohumeral, 3 cervical facet, and 2 hip joints that received intra-articular injections. Treated tendons included 7 common extensor tendons at the elbow, 3 supraspinatus, 3 conjoint hamstring, 2 gluteus medius, 2 patellar, 1 Achilles tendon, 1 peroneus longus, and 1 iliopsoas. Despite a transient increase in pain at the injection site that lasted an average of 2 days, significant improvements in patient's pain and function at 1, 2, and 3 months of follow-up were reported.

Vines and colleagues[48] performed an open-label prospective pilot study to determine the feasibility and safety of injection of a cryopreserved particulated human AM and AF (ReNu; Organogenesis Inc, Canton, MA, USA) for the treatment of symptomatic knee osteoarthritis. Patients were assessed before treatment and at 1 and 2 weeks, and 3, 6, and 12 months after treatment. Safety was assessed by physical examination and laboratory data. Although statistical significance was not achieved due to the small sample size, there was a general trend toward improvement in all patient-reported outcomes. There was a statistically significant increase in immunoglobulin G and E levels in approximately 15% of the samples at the 12-month time point; however, these levels were still considered within normal reference ranges. Two adverse events were reported with 2 patients experiencing a transient increase in pain after the injection, which resolved by the 2-week follow-up. In summary, injections were well tolerated, indicating the feasibility of a single intra-articular injection of ASA for the treatment of symptomatic knee osteoarthritis. A large, multicenter, placebo-controlled trial is currently under way.

A query of clinicaltrials.gov in February 2018 identified 18 ongoing clinical trials for the use of amniotic-derived products for orthopedic sports medicine applications. These studies include injectable products for the treatment of osteoarthritis, plantar fasciitis, and Achilles tendonitis, and also as augmentation in the surgical treatment of rotator cuff tears, ACL injury, articular cartilage defects, and peroneal and Achilles tendon injury.

SUMMARY

Amniotic-derived products in sports medicine are a rapidly expanding area in orthobiologics with several preclinical studies showing promising results. However, small sample sizes and short follow-up limit the conclusions that can be drawn from the current literature for clinical use in humans. Despite the proven safety of amniotic-derived products, the efficacy and mechanisms by which they exert a therapeutic benefit are unknown. Current commercially available products are typically acellular or have limited cell viability due to processing, sterilization, and storage methods. Therefore, it is likely that AM-derived products deliver a therapeutic benefit through their intrinsic properties as an extracellular matrix, and the presence of growth factors, anti-inflammatory, antimicrobial, and antifibrotic molecules.

Not all amniotic-derived products are created equal, and it is important to understand the harvesting, processing, sterilization, and storage methods of each individual product. Although these products do not share the same ethical concerns as embryonic-derived MSCs, some patients may have personal or religious objections to their use, and it is the responsibility of the clinician to help patients make informed decisions about using these products. In addition, essentially all insurance companies consider these products investigational and therefore do not cover their use, which can lead to a substantial "out-of-pocket" cost to the patient. As this area of orthobiologics is advancing, it will be important for clinicians to understand the individual products, and for higher-quality clinical trials to further elucidate their specific applications, therapeutic benefit, and cost-effectiveness.

REFERENCES

1. Caplan AI. Adult mesenchymal stem cells for tissue engineering versus regenerative medicine. J Cell Physiol 2007;213(2):341–7.
2. De Bari C, Dell'Accio F, Tylzanowski P, et al. Multipotent mesenchymal stem cells from adult human synovial membrane. Arthritis Rheum 2001;44(8):1928–42.
3. Zuk PA, Zhu M, Ashjian P, et al. Human adipose tissue is a source of multipotent stem cells. Mol Biol Cell 2002;13(12):4279–95.
4. Nishida S, Endo N, Yamagiwa H, et al. Number of osteoprogenitor cells in human bone marrow markedly decreases after skeletal maturation. J Bone Miner Metab 1999;17(3):171–7.
5. Oliver K, Awan T, Bayes M. Single- versus multiple-site harvesting techniques for bone marrow concentrate: evaluation of aspirate quality and pain. Orthop J Sport Med 2017;5(8). 2325967117724398.
6. Baghaban Eslaminejad M, Jahangir S. Amniotic fluid stem cells and their application in cell-based tissue regeneration. Int J Fertil Steril 2012;6(3):147–56.
7. Riboh JC, Saltzman BM, Yanke AB, et al. Human amniotic membrane–derived products in sports medicine. Am J Sports Med 2016;44(9):2425–34.
8. Niknejad H, Peirovi H, Jorjani M, et al. Properties of the amniotic membrane for potential use in tissue engineering. Eur Cell Mater 2008;15:88–99.

9. Pollard SM, Aye NN, Symonds EM. Scanning electron microscope appearances of normal human amnion and umbilical cord at term. Br J Obstet Gynaecol 1976; 83(6):470–7.
10. Rocha SCM, Baptista CJM. Biochemical properties of amniotic membrane. In: amniotic membrane. Dordrecht (Netherlands): Springer Netherlands; 2015. p. 19–40.
11. Fairbairn NG, Randolph MA, Redmond RW. The clinical applications of human amnion in plastic surgery. J Plast Reconstr Aesthet Surg 2014;67(5):662–75.
12. Okroj M, Holmquist E, Sjölander J, et al. Heavy chains of inter alpha inhibitor (IαI) inhibit the human complement system at early stages of the cascade. J Biol Chem 2012;287(24):20100–10.
13. Kim JS, Kim JC, Na BK, et al. Amniotic membrane patching promotes healing and inhibits proteinase activity on wound healing following acute corneal alkali burn. Exp Eye Res 2000;70(3):329–37.
14. King AE, Paltoo A, Kelly RW, et al. Expression of natural antimicrobials by human placenta and fetal membranes. Placenta 2007;28(2–3):161–9.
15. Le Blanc K, Tammik C, Rosendahl K, et al. HLA expression and immunologic properties of differentiated and undifferentiated mesenchymal stem cells. Exp Hematol 2003;31(10):890–6.
16. Friel NA, De Girolamo L, Gomoll AH, et al. Amniotic fluid, cells, and membrane application. Oper Tech Sports Med 2017;25(1):20–4.
17. McIntyre JA, Jones IA, Danilkovich A, et al. The placenta applications in orthopaedic sports medicine. Am J Sports Med 2018;46(1):234–47.
18. Malhotra C, Jain AK. Human amniotic membrane transplantation: different modalities of its use in ophthalmology. World J Transplant 2014;4(2):111–21.
19. Niknejad H, Deihim T, Solati-Hashjin M, et al. The effects of preservation procedures on amniotic membrane's ability to serve as a substrate for cultivation of endothelial cells. Cryobiology 2011;63(3):145–51.
20. McQuilling JP, Vines JB, Kimmerling KA, et al. Proteomic comparison of amnion and chorion and evaluation of the effects of processing on placental membranes. Wounds 2017;29(6):E38–42.
21. Nogami M, Kimura T, Seki S, et al. A human amnion-derived extracellular matrix-coated cell-free scaffold for cartilage repair: in vitro and in vivo studies. Tissue Eng Part A 2016;22(7–8):680–8.
22. Wei JP, Nawata M, Wakitani S, et al. Human amniotic mesenchymal cells differentiate into chondrocytes. Cloning Stem Cells 2009;11(1):19–26.
23. Garcia D, Longo UG, Vaquero J, et al. Amniotic membrane transplant for articular cartilage repair: an experimental study in sheep. Curr Stem Cell Res Ther 2015; 10(1):77–83.
24. Tabet SK, Conner DM, Guebert DA. The use of human amniotic membrane for cartilage repair: a sheep study. Stem Cell Discov 2015;5(4):40–7.
25. Jin CZ, Park SR, Choi BH, et al. Human amniotic membrane as a delivery matrix for articular cartilage repair. Tissue Eng 2007;13(4):693–702.
26. Willett NJ, Thote T, Lin ASP, et al. Intra-articular injection of micronized dehydrated human amnion/chorion membrane attenuates osteoarthritis development. Arthritis Res Ther 2014;16(1):R47.
27. Kim J, Kim T, Park S, et al. Protective effects of human placenta extract on cartilage degradation in experimental osteoarthritis. Biol Pharm Bull 2010;33(6): 1004–10.
28. Coban I, Satoğlu IS, Gültekin A, et al. Effects of human amniotic fluid and membrane in the treatment of Achilles tendon ruptures in locally corticosteroid-

induced Achilles tendinosis: an experimental study on rats. Foot Ankle Surg 2009;15(1):22–7.

29. Muttini A, Mattioli M, Petrizzi L, et al. Experimental study on allografts of amniotic epithelial cells in calcaneal tendon lesions of sheep. Vet Res Commun 2010; 34(S1):117–20.

30. Barboni B, Russo V, Curini V, et al. Achilles tendon regeneration can be improved by amniotic epithelial cell allotransplantation. Cell Transplant 2012;21(11): 2377–95.

31. Steed DL, Trumpower C, Duffy D, et al. Amnion-derived cellular cytokine solution: a physiological combination of cytokines for wound healing. Eplasty 2008;8:e18.

32. Philip J, Hackl F, Canseco JA, et al. Amnion-derived multipotent progenitor cells improve achilles tendon repair in rats. Eplasty 2013;13:e31.

33. Kueckelhaus M, Philip J, Kamel RA, et al. Sustained release of amnion-derived cellular cytokine solution facilitates achilles tendon healing in rats. Eplasty 2014;14:e29.

34. Ozgenel GY. The effects of a combination of hyaluronic and amniotic membrane on the formation of peritendinous adhesions after flexor tendon surgery in chickens. J Bone Joint Surg Br 2004;86(2):301–7.

35. Özgenel GY, Şamli B, Özcan M. Effects of human amniotic fluid on peritendinous adhesion formation and tendon healing after flexor tendon surgery in rabbits. J Hand Surg Am 2001;26(2):332–9.

36. Özbölük Ş, Özkan Y, Öztürk A, et al. The effects of human amniotic membrane and periosteal autograft on tendon healing: experimental study in rabbits. J Hand Surg Eur Vol 2010;35(4):262–8.

37. Demirkan F, Colakoglu N, Herek O, et al. The use of amniotic membrane in flexor tendon repair: an experimental model. Arch Orthop Trauma Surg 2002;122(7): 396–9.

38. Muttini A, Valbonetti L, Abate M, et al. Ovine amniotic epithelial cells: in vitro characterization and transplantation into equine superficial digital flexor tendon spontaneous defects. Res Vet Sci 2013;94(1):158–69.

39. Muttini A, Russo V, Rossi E, et al. Pilot experimental study on amniotic epithelial mesenchymal cell transplantation in natural occurring tendinopathy in horses. Ultrasonographic and histological comparison. Muscles Ligaments Tendons J 2015;5(1):5–11.

40. Lange-Consiglio A, Tassan S, Corradetti B, et al. Investigating the efficacy of amnion-derived compared with bone marrow–derived mesenchymal stromal cells in equine tendon and ligament injuries. Cytotherapy 2013;15(8):1011–20.

41. Lange-Consiglio A, Rossi D, Tassan S, et al. Conditioned medium from horse amniotic membrane-derived multipotent progenitor cells: immunomodulatory activity in vitro and first clinical application in tendon and ligament injuries in vivo. Stem Cells Dev 2013;22(22):3015–24.

42. Hanselman AE, Tidwell JE, Santrock RD. Cryopreserved human amniotic membrane injection for plantar fasciitis. Foot Ankle Int 2015;36(2):151–8.

43. Zelen CM, Poka A, Andrews J. Prospective, randomized, blinded, comparative study of injectable micronized dehydrated amniotic/chorionic membrane allograft for plantar fasciitis - a feasibility study. Foot Ankle Int 2013;34(10):1332–9.

44. Werber B. Amniotic tissues for the treatment of chronic plantar fasciosis and achilles tendinosis. J Sport Med (Hindawi Publ Corp) 2015;2015:219896.

45. Lullove E. A flowable placental tissue matrix allograft in lower extremity injuries: a pilot study. Cureus 2015;7(6):e275.

46. Warner M, Lasyone L. An open-label, single-center, retrospective study of cryo-preserved amniotic membrane and umbilical cord tissue as an adjunct for foot and ankle surgery. Surg Technol Int 2014;25:251–5.

47. Gellhorn AC, Han A. The use of dehydrated human amnion/chorion membrane allograft injection for the treatment of tendinopathy or arthritis: a case series involving 40 patients. PM R 2017;9(12):1236–43.

48. Vines J, Aliprantis A, Gomoll A, et al. Cryopreserved amniotic suspension for the treatment of knee osteoarthritis. J Knee Surg 2015;29(6):443–50.

Adipose-Derived Stem Cell Treatments and Formulations

Berardo Di Matteo, MD[a,b,*], Mohamed Marzouk El Araby, MD[a,b],
Alessandro D'Angelo, MD[c], Francesco Iacono, MD[a,b], Alessandra Nannini, MD[a,b],
Nicolò Danilo Vitale, MD[a,b], Maurilio Marcacci, MD[a,b], Stefano Respizzi, MD[a,b],
Elizaveta Kon, MD[a,b]

KEYWORDS

- Stem cells • Adipose-derived mesenchymal stem cells • Stromal vascular fraction
- Intra-articular injection • Cartilage • Osteoarthritis

KEY POINTS

- In vitro and animal trials have shown that adipose-derived stem cells (ASCs) are able to exert immune-modulatory and trophic effects on the articular environment.
- The available evidence on the clinical application of ASCs is lacking high-quality clinical trials to clarify the best applicative modalities and therapeutic protocols.
- The most widely adopted strategy in the clinical setting relies on the intra-articular injection of the stromal vascular fraction (SVF) obtained from the lipoaspirate.
- Based on the available evidence, no significant difference in efficacy has been reported between SVF and expanded cells.
- The overall clinical results seem promising at short-term evaluation, although ASCs are often used together with other biologic products, thus making it difficult to identify the true potential of the cells.

INTRODUCTION

Many pharmacologic and surgical approaches have been proposed in the past years for the treatment of cartilage pathology.[1] The alteration of the articular surface, such as with osteoarthritis (OA) or a focal cartilage defect, is perceived by the patient both as pain as well as dysfunction of the joint. The loss of the functional properties of cartilage leads to pathologic modification of the subchondral bone and progressive articular

Disclosure Statement: All the authors of the present article have nothing to disclose.
Funding Source Statement: No funding source to be declared for the present article.
[a] Department of Biomedical Sciences, Humanitas University, Via Manzoni 113, Rozzano, Milan 20089, Italy; [b] Humanitas Clinical and Research Center, Via Manzoni 56, Rozzano, Milan 20089, Italy; [c] Department of Orthopaedic, Traumatology and Rehabilitation, Azienda Ospedaliero Universitaria Città della Salute e della Scienza, CTO Hospital, Via Zuretti 29, Turin 10126, Italy
* Corresponding author. Humanitas Clinical and Research Center, Via Manzoni 56, Rozzano, Milan 20089, Italy.
E-mail address: berardo.dimatteo@gmail.com

degeneration, resulting in OA.[2] Young patients with OA are a challenging population due to the combination of their high functional demands and limited indications for invasive surgical treatments. Today, the same can be said for middle-aged active patients who often want to maintain a high level of activity and postpone or avoid metal resurfacing. Despite the rising incidence of OA, currently, there are no effective therapies to restore the original features and structure of the damaged articular surface. Regenerative scaffold-based procedures are emerging as a promising therapeutic option for the treatment of chondral lesions with the aim of regenerating hyaline cartilage,[3] but, even if short-term results are promising, current evidence is lacking in long-term results.[4] Thus far, no surgical technique has been completely successful in stimulating cartilage regeneration and/or repair. Conservative or minimally invasive treatments currently available aim to improve the symptomatology of the patient, but their ability to regenerate the damaged area is unclear.

Looking for a new direction in cartilage regeneration, innovative therapies have been introduced. These have ranged from platelet-derived growth factors to cell-based treatments and have also been combined with various biomaterials for tissue engineering strategies.[5,6] Mesenchymal stem cells (MSCs) have emerged as a valid alternative to the use of differentiated chondrocytes. Thanks to their multilineage differentiation potential and multipotency, they are able to differentiate into several lines, such as osteoblasts, chondrocytes, myoblasts, or adipocytes. MSCs also have high plasticity, immune-suppressive and anti-inflammatory actions, and the capability of self-renewal.[7] Growth factors, cytokines, bioactive lipids, and microvesicles released from stem cells may also exert beneficial effects, including angiopoietic and antiapoptotic actions. Therefore, the observed improvements in pain relief and joint function after MSC injection may in fact be due to the paracrine effects of MSCs, perhaps suggesting that the biologic agents secreted by stem cells, rather than the cells themselves, act as the therapeutic agents.

Subsequent studies have highlighted the presence of MSCs in numerous adult tissues, including adipose, muscle, dermis, periosteum, synovial membrane, synovial fluid, and articular cartilage.[8] Choosing the right stem cell approach is imperative for obtaining favorable results in regenerative medicine. Among these sources, adipose-derived mesenchymal stem cells (ASCs) are attracting attention as an alternative to the "traditional" and more studied bone marrow mesenchymal stem cells (BMSCs).[9,10]

Since the first case report in 2011, ASCs have demonstrated safety and efficacy for articular cartilage regeneration in several phase I/II clinical trials. It has been shown that the immunophenotypes of BMSCs and ASCs are more than 90% identical[11,12]; however, some minor differences seem to exist, as they exhibit a number of distinct characteristics, such as their cell surface markers, differentiation potential, and distribution in the body. The greatest advantage of ASCs is their abundance: when compared with 100 mL of bone marrow aspirate, up to 300-fold more stem cells can be obtained from 100 g of adipose tissue.[13,14]

Other advantages include the ease of harvesting with low donor-site morbidity and the rapid expansion and high proliferation potential of these cells.[12] Moreover, it has been shown that ASCs can maintain their phenotype better over many culture passages as compared with BMSCs[15] Specifically, human ASCs are more genetically and morphologically stable in a long-term culture,[16] display a lower senescence ratio, and show a higher proliferative capacity.[16,17] A recent study clearly demonstrated that human ASCs support hematopoiesis both in vitro and in vivo and, unexpectedly, seem to exert this activity more efficiently than human BMSCs.[18]

Over the past decade, the number of preclinical and clinical studies dealing with ASCs has increased significantly; however, their mechanism of action is still not fully understood. Both the differentiation process of stem cells as well as their paracrine and trophic effects are still under investigation. Moreover, the optimal strategy for the clinical application of ASCs has not yet been identified, and many aspects still remain controversial.[19] The aim of this systematic review is to analyze the current literature on the use of ASCs in the clinical setting to show the available evidence regarding their therapeutic potential for cartilage regeneration and to understand possible future application strategies for the treatment of chondral pathologies.

MATERIALS AND METHODS

A systematic review of the literature was performed on the use of ASCs for OA or cartilage defects in vivo. The guidelines for Preferred Reporting Items for Systematic Reviews and Meta-analysis (PRISMA) were used. Screening process and analysis were conducted separately by 3 independent observers (MMEA, ADA, NDV). The search was performed on the PubMed database, focusing on clinical studies with the following thread: "cartilage" OR "osteoarthritis" AND "adipose-derived mesenchymal stem cells" OR "adipose-derived stem cells" OR "adipose derived stromal cells" OR "stromal vascular fraction" OR "SVF" OR "ASC" OR "ASCs." The filters included publications from the past 15 years in the English language. Articles were first screened by title and abstract. Reference lists were also screened to obtain further studies for this review. Articles were then carefully analyzed, and those not reporting the in vivo use of ASCs or reporting applications different from cartilage defects or OA were excluded. Relevant data were then extracted and collected in a unique database with the consensus of the 2 observers to be analyzed for the purposes of the present article. Based on the finding that the vast majority of the clinical trials identified focused on knee pathology and few studies investigated ASCs in other joints, the present review was oriented toward the analysis of results concerning knee cartilage pathology.

RESULTS

A total of 1030 articles were screened according to the aforementioned inclusion criteria, and 18 were included in the analysis. One article was withdrawn by the publisher during the production of this review, so it was excluded, leading to a final number of 17 articles undergoing analysis for the present article (**Fig. 1**).[20–36] A detailed description of each study is provided in **Table 1**. Looking at the quality of the trials, only 5 of 17 were comparative. In 1 study, 2 different application methods of ASCs were compared: local adhesion of ASCs onto the defect versus delivery through a fibrin glue addition. Two studies tested ASCs at different dosages to determine if a correlation was present between dose and clinical response. In the fourth comparative study, ASC injections were given as adjunctive treatment to patients undergoing high tibial osteotomy with or without the subsequent addition of platelet-rich plasma (PRP). In the final comparative study analyzed for this review, injection of ASCs + PRP was tested against PRP alone.

The most common harvest site for ASCs was the abdominal area, followed by the buttocks. In all cases, ASCs were administered by intra-articular injection; in 5 studies, the injection was preceded by arthroscopic debridement (4) or high tibial osteotomy (1). The average number of patients included was low in the vast majority of cases, with only 3 trials including at least 50 patients. The follow-up evaluation reached 24 months or more in just 6 of 17 studies, whereas the remaining trials reported results at shorter evaluation, mainly 6 and 12 months of follow-up.

With regard to the formulations, 14 cases used the stromal vascular fraction (SVF), that is, concentrated ASCs without cell culture. The most common preparation method for SVF consisted of the use of collagenase to digest the lipoaspirate, followed

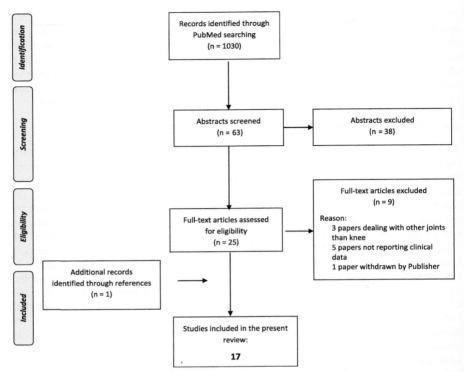

Fig. 1. Flowchart showing the selection process of articles for the present review.

by centrifugation to remove the enzymatic portion and to further concentrate the ASCs before their intra-articular delivery. In the remaining 3 studies, expanded ASCs were used, indicating that a 2-step procedure was performed on patients.

In 11 trials, ASCs were applied with other agents, including PRP, PRP + hyaluronic acid (HA), or even PRP + HA + dexamethasone, thus clouding the identification of the true contribution of ASCs in terms of clinical effectiveness. In some cases, the application of ASCs, with or without other biologic products, was followed by further injections in the postoperative period. In all cases, these additional injections included PRP and/or HA.

In terms of clinical results, no major adverse events were reported after the application of ASCs, and overall encouraging clinical findings were reported, with an increase in functional subjective scores and pain reduction. Poor radiologic data were collected in 6 studies, and so it is difficult to offer a reliable evaluation in this particular field of analysis. Although second-look arthroscopies were performed in a few cases, limiting the relevance of the data, better arthroscopic appearance of the cartilage was observed in the treated joints. The most interesting findings were reported by Koh and colleagues,[29] who performed second-look arthroscopies at the time of hardware removal in patients previously treated with high tibial osteotomy and injection of either ASC + PRP or PRP alone. This study found significantly better cartilage repair in the ASC + PRP group when compared with the PRP group alone.

Interestingly, the 2 trials[27,32] compared varying doses of ASCs, both of which used expanded cells, revealed contrasting results. In one study, only the high-dose regimen was able to produce significant clinical improvement, whereas the other study

Table 1
Synopsis of the clinical trials included in the present systematic review dealing with the application of ASCs in cartilage pathology

Reference	Study Design	Pathology	Cell Type and Source	Methods for Obtaining ASCs	Application Modality	Treatment Protocol	Number of Patients	Follow-up	Results
Pak et al,[20] 2011	Case report	Knee OA	SVF Abdominal area	Adipose tissue centrifuged for 5 min, digested for 30 min at 37° with an equal volume of digestive enzyme (0.07% collagenase type 1) and centrifuged at 100g for 3 min to separate the lipoaspirate and enzyme. After removing the leftover enzyme, the lipoaspirate was washed 3 times using 5% dextrose in lactate Ringer solution and centrifuged 3 times at 100g.	Single injection	i. ASCs + PRP + HA + dexamethasone	2	3 mo	Cartilage volume increased at MRI Improved functional status
Koh & Choi,[21] 2012	Comparative study	Knee OA	SVF Infrapatellar fad pad	Lipoaspirates digested with 0.1% collagenase type 1, incubated at 37°C with continuous agitation for 3 h and subsequently centrifuged at 1200g for 10 min to separate the lipoaspirate from the collagenase; finally, the lipoaspirate was washed 3 times to remove any remaining collagenase	Single injection after debridement	i. ASCs + PRP ii. Only PRP (control)	Study group: 25 Control group: 25	16.4 mo	Significant improvement in all clinical scores. Study vs control: n.s. at final follow-up, but study group had lower basal

(continued on next page)

Table 1
(*continued*)

Reference	Study Design	Pathology	Cell Type and Source	Methods for Obtaining ASCs	Application Modality	Treatment Protocol	Number of Patients	Follow-up	Results
Pak et al,[22] 2013	Case series	Knee OA	SVF Abdominal area	Lipoaspirates digested with an equal volume of digestive enzyme (0.07% collagenase type 1) for 30 min at 37°C and then centrifuged at 100g for 3 min to separate the lipoaspirate and the enzyme. Finally washed using 5% dextrose in lactate Ringer solution and centrifuged, after each washing, at 100g 3 times, to remove collagenase	Single injection	i. ASCs + PRP + HA	91	30 mo	VAS improved 50%–60% No major complications
Pak et al,[23] 2013	Case series	Chondromalacia patellae	SVF Abdominal area	Lipoaspirates digested with 0.07% collagenase type 1 and centrifuged at 500g	Single injection	i. ASCs + PRP + HA	3	12 mo	Pain improved: 50%–70% at 1 m 80%–90% at 3 m
Koh et al,[24] 2013	Case series	Knee OA	SVF Buttocks	Lipoaspirates digested with 0.075% collagenase for 30 min at 37°C; enzyme activity neutralized with DMEM; after obtaining a high-density SVF pellet trough centrifugation at 1200g for 10 min, the pellet itself was resuspended in 160 mM NH4Cl and incubated at room temperature for 10 min to lyse contaminating RBCs	Single injection	i. ASCs + PRP	30	24 mo	Significant clinical improvement 14/16 (87.5%) of 2nd look arthroscopy within 24 m improved or maintained cartilage status Further clinical improvement 24 vs 12m

Koh et al,[25] 2013	Case series	Knee OA	SVF Infrapatellar fat pad	Lipoaspirates digested with 0.1% collagenase type 1, incubated at 37°C with continuous agitation for 3 h and subsequently centrifuged at 1200g for 10 min to separate the lipoaspirate from the collagenase; finally the lipoaspirate was washed 3 times to remove any remaining collagenase	Single injection after debridement	i. ASCs + PRP	18	24.3 mo	Significant improvement of the clinical and MRI scores at final follow-up
Bui et al,[26] 2014	Case series	Knee OA	SVF Abdominal area	Lipoaspirates centrifuged at 400g for 5 min at room temperature, then digested with collagenase for 30 min at 37°C with agitation at 5-min intervals; the suspension is then centrifuged at 800g for 10 min, gaining a pellet that was washed twice with PBS to remove any residual enzyme	Single injection	i. ASCs + PRP	21	6 mo	Function improvement in all patients at 8.5 m; Increased cartilage thickness on MRI
Jo et al,[27] 2014	Comparative trial + case series	Knee OA	Expanded Abdominal area	Lipoaspirates digested under agitation with 0.075% collagenase for 60 min at 37°C then filtered through a 100-mm nylon to obtain a pellet that is suspended in a DMEM and subsequently centrifuged at 470g for 5 min	Single injection	i. Phase I: 3 doses of ASCs; the low-, mid-, and high-dose group with 3 patients each; ii. Phase II: 9 patients receiving the high dose of ASCs	18	6 mo	Clinical improvement and hyalinelike regenerative tissue only in high-dose group, without adverse events

(continued on next page)

Table 1
(continued)

Reference	Study Design	Pathology	Cell Type and Source	Methods for Obtaining ASCs	Application Modality	Treatment Protocol	Number of Patients	Follow-up	Results
Koh et al,[28] 2014	Case series	Knee OA	SVF Buttocks	Lipoaspirates digested with 0.075% collagenase for 30 min at 37°C; enzyme activity neutralized with DMEM; after obtaining a high-density SVF pellet through centrifugation at 1200g for 10 min, the pellet itself is resuspended in 160 mM NH4Cl and incubated at room temperature for 10 min to lyse contaminating RBCs	Single injection after debridement	i. ASCs local adherent technique	35 (37 knees)	12.7 mo	Clinical improvement; 94% patients excellent or good satisfaction 76% abnormal or severely abnormal repair tissue at 2nd look
Koh et al,[29] 2014	Comparative study	Knee OA	SVF Buttocks	Same as above	Single injection after debridement	i. HTO + PRP + ASCs (= 23) ii. HTO + PRP (= 21)	44	24 mo	Better clinical improvement in PRP + ADSCs group (some KOOS subgroups) Better tissue healing at second look for PRP + ADSCs
Kim et al,[30] 2015	Comparative study	Knee OA	SVF Buttocks	Same as above	Single injection after debridement	i. ASCs local adherent (= 37) ii. ASCs on FG (= 17)	54 (56 knees) Second look	28.6 m 12.3 m (second look)	Overall clinical improvement Comparable for both groups Better ICRS scores at second look for ADSC-FG group Lower BMI and smaller size positively correlate with outcomes

Gibbs,[31] 2015	Case series	Knee OA	SVF abdominal area	100 mL of lipoaspirate collected in 4 syringes; lipoaspirate was processed using the Cell-Innovations Pty Ltd ultrasonic cavitation protocol; the cell solution was filtered through a 100-μm filter and pellet resuspended in 0.9% saline	Single injection of ADSC + PRP, plus only PRP injection 2-3-4 mo	i. ASCs + PRP + exercise (4-mo supervised progressive resistance training program incorporating specific water and land-based exercises)	4 (7 knees)	12 mo	All patients demonstrated improvement in knee-related QOL and KOOS subscales
Pers,[32] 2016	Clinical trial (phase 1)	Knee OA	Cultured AD-MSCs abdominal area	10 g of adipose tissue were mixed with 34 mL collagenase solution and incubated at 37°C for 45 min, then added with human platelet growth factor-enriched plasma, 10 mg/mL ciprofloxacin, and 1 U/mL heparin; the suspension was passed through 100-mm filters; the cells were centrifuged at room temperature for 10 min at 600g and seeded	Single injection	ASC at 3 different concentrations: i. Low dose (2×10^6) ii. Medium 10×10^6 iii. High dose (50×10^6)	18	6 mo	Improvement for all clinical outcome parameters (pain, function, and mobility) regardless of the injected dose; possible cartilage improvement in 3 of 6 patients
Fodor,[33] 2016	Case series	Knee OA	SVF abdominal area, flanks, lateral thighs	Lipoaspirate disaggregated using Type I collagenase at a concentration of 200 CDU/mL in equal volume of 37°C LR solution; incubated in shaker for 40 min at 38°C at 150 revolutions/min; added human albumin 2.5%; the device was then centrifuged at 800g for 10 min	Single injection	i. ASCs	6 (8 knees)	12 mo	Statistically significant improvement in WOMAC and VAS score; no detectable structural differences at MRI assessment from preoperative time to 3-mo postoperative measurements

(continued on next page)

Table 1 (continued)							
Reference	Study Design	Pathology	Cell Type and Source	Methods for Obtaining ASCs	Application Modality	Treatment Protocol	Number of Patients	Follow-up	Results
Pak et al,[34] 2016	Case series	Knee OA	SVF abdominal area	Lipoaspirate 50 mL centrifuged at 1600g for 5 min, homogenized 40 times; digested by collagenase type I 0.07% at 37°C for 40 min; centrifuged at 330g to separate and remove collagenase solution; saline + dextrose 5% up to 50 mL, and centrifugated again	Single injection + 3 injection of HA + PRP	i. ASCs + PRP + HA	3.	3 mo	All clinical criteria of FRI, VAS score, and ROM improved in all patients, along with significant MRI change
Spasovski et al,[35] 2017	Case series	Knee OA	Cultured AD-MSCs abdominal area	Lipoaspirate of 5 mL, washed in 1× PBS solution, digested with 0.1% collagenase; centrifugation for 10 min; filtered through 0.22 μm; collagenase solution was neutralized by low glucose and filtered through 100-μm filter, counted and seeded in number of $6 \times 10^4/cm^2$ in DMEM/10% autologous serum/1X antibiotic/antimycotic; after 1 wk, floating cells were washed away and cultured for 2–3 wk, until they reached number of $0.5{-}1.0 \times 10^7$	Single injection	i. ASCs	9 (11 knees)	18 mo	Significant improvement of all clinical score applied (KSS, HSS-KS, VAS score) Significant cartilage restoration at MOCART score, while no improvement at radiographs

Bansal et al,[36] 2017	Case series	Knee OA	SVF abdominal area	Lipoaspirate 100 mL digested using collagenase for 30 min 37°C, centrifuged at 500g for 5 min; any residual enzyme was removed and filtered through 100 μm; the cells were washed twice and centrifuged for 10 min; supernatant was discarded; the pellet was resuspended in complete DMEM (Sigma) and plated in a T25 flask and incubated at 37°C under 5% CO_2; medium was changed every 3–4 d until the cells achieved 90% confluency	Single injection	i. ASCs + PRP	10. (13 knees)	24 mo	Both qualitative and quantitative measurements showed statistically significant improvement (WOMAC, XR, MRI)

Abbreviations: ASCs, adipose-derived stem cells; BMI, body mass index; DMEM, Dulbecco modified Eagle medium; FG, fibrin glue; FRI, functional rating index; HA, hyaluronic acid; HSS-KS, hospital for special surgery knee score; HTO, high tibial osteotomy; ICRS, international cartilage repair society; KOOS, knee injury and osteoarthritis outcome score; KSS, knee society score; LR, lactate Ringer; MOCART, magnetic resonance observation of cartilage repair tissue; ns, not significant; OA, osteoarthritis; PBS, phosphate-buffered saline; PRP, platelet-rich plasma; QOL, quality of life; RBC, red blood cell; ROM, range of motion; SVF, stromal vascular fraction; T-L, tegner-lysholm; VAS, visual analog scale; WOMAC, Western Ontario and McMaster Universities Osteoarthritis Index; XR, x-rays.

observed no intergroup difference, and clinical improvement occurred independently from the dose of ASCs administered.

DISCUSSION

The main finding of this review is that there remains little high-quality evidence supporting the efficacy of adipose-derived MSCs for the treatment of knee articular degeneration. Most studies are case series with follow-up limited to short-term evaluation with a relatively small number of patients included. Furthermore, there are no clear indications on the best processing strategies, therapeutic protocols, application modalities, or dosages to be used in clinical practice to maximize clinical outcomes. Based on the current available literature, the use of ASCs appears to be safe with encouraging clinical results in terms of functional recovery and pain reduction, suggesting that this biologic approach might play a promising role as a minimally invasive treatment option for OA. Further studies, both in vitro and in vivo, will help to elucidate the true potential of this novel approach.

Overall, MSCs are a well-characterized population of tissue-resident adult stem cells. They are present in many tissues and organs within specific cell niches, where they colocalize with supporting cells.[37] MSCs fulfill a critical role in the maintenance of homeostasis by replenishing the mature cell types within the tissues in which they reside over a person's lifetime. The current trend is to use these MSCs to replenish mature cell types within other tissues as well. Particularly, ASCs are currently being used in clinical settings for various applications in humans, including a wide spectrum of musculoskeletal conditions. Due to their potential capability of regenerating cartilage and bone, ASCs are being applied in the treatment of rheumatoid arthritis (RA), osteoarthritis, chondromalacia, and osteonecrosis of the femoral head.[34]

In patients with RA, ASCs have shown therapeutic effects in vitro.[38] They inhibit T-cell proliferation, produce cytokines, and generate antigen-specific regulatory T cells. Thus, they suppress the responses of collagen II–reactive T cells in patients with RA. In a recent study, Álvaro-Gracia and colleagues[39] evaluated the safety and tolerability of the intravenous administration of ASCs, documenting their safety and the absence of dose-related toxicity. Intra-articular injections of ASCs have been shown to reduce synovitis, osteophyte formation, and cartilage degeneration in animal models[40,41] of OA as well as of focal osteochondral defects.[42]

The wide range of actions of these multipotent cells is able to provide both a modulation of the intra-articular environment, delaying the progression of degenerative changes, and a positive effect on the regeneration of hyaline cartilage when used in the treatment of isolated cartilage lesions in adjunct to biomaterials. Looking at the animal literature, most trials have studied expanded ASCs, which is in contrast to current clinical literature, in which the predominant use is of nonexpanded ASCs, that is, the so-called SVF. The SVF consists of a "tissue niche" containing a variety of stem cells, progenitor cells, and adult cells, all of which could potentially play a beneficial role in cartilage healing and repair. Approximately 10% of the cells of the SVF have been identified as ASCs.[6] Despite this unfavorable ratio compared with cultured cells, current in vitro and in vivo literature has shown no significant differences between expanded ASCs and SVF. Of note, one report documented superior cartilage regeneration using SVF as compared with expanded cells.[43] This finding is of particular translational relevance, as cell expansion is subject to higher processing costs and stricter regulatory issues in many countries, thus making its adoption problematic on many levels. Conversely, the use of SVF, which is a "single-step" procedure in which the lipoaspirate can be immediately processed in the operating room and applied in the joint, is a much more physician-friendly and patient-friendly method, justifying its larger use in the clinical setting and use in most clinical trials currently available.

For preparation, mechanical, enzymatic, and combined processing methods have been proposed, often accompanied by one or multiple centrifugations at different speeds. Thus, it is still impossible to endorse a specific method over the others.[20–26] Nevertheless, the promising clinical results obtained with SVF make this method the easiest and most suitable way to exploit ASCs in humans. Still, further studies are needed to clarify whether cellular expansion could provide superior efficacy in the treatment of cartilage pathology.

As often happens with biologic products, a wide variability in product preparation, therapeutic protocol, timing of application, and concurrent treatments has been documented, thus jeopardizing interstudy comparability.[42] The most widely adopted delivery method in humans is an intra-articular injection. This can be performed without additional surgical intervention, with some investigators preferring to apply ASCs without previous arthroscopic inspection to avoid surgical distress on the joint, which could impair the overall effect of stem cells. Others instead are using ASCs as an "augmentation" after debridement or more complex procedures such as osteotomy,[29] with the aim of improving clinical outcomes. In one trial, investigators tested ASCs in the treatment of focal chondral defects and compared the results of 2 different application modalities: direct adhesion of cells to the lesion and adhesion through the addition of fibrin glue.[30] The limited amount of data available prevents the establishment of the optimal treatment approach at the moment.

Additionally, stem cells could be exploited in several other ways, such as an additional enhancement after microfracture or within membranes or biomaterials to create a cellularized scaffold for the treatment of chondral/osteochondral defects.[44] Their versatility is both an advantage and a limiting factor, due to the inherent difficulties in assessing and understanding the true contribution of ASCs alone. Currently, this is the major issue clinicians have to face when dealing with the results of ASCs application. The present review showed that in most cases, ASCs were used together with other biologically active products, particularly PRP, the contribution of which cannot be underestimated.[45] Unfortunately, there is only one comparative trial analyzing injection of ASCs + PRP versus PRP alone,[21] but findings were inconclusive. Thus, further randomized controlled trials must be completed to more clearly demonstrate the clinical potential of ASCs. Perhaps the combination of ASCs with other biologic agents will increase the overall efficacy and maximize results, but more evidence is needed before any indiscriminate use of these products. Similar consideration can be raised regarding the combination of ASCs and biomaterials, which has been evaluated in many animal trials.[46,47] Overall, the ASCs seemed to provide a beneficial contribution in terms of tissue healing and maturation with different biomaterials, but these results must be still confirmed in the human setting. As seen in the past, there is a tendency to push the use of multiple biologic products in clinical practice without understanding high-quality clinical research. The result is that the quest for the best outcome is often slowing down (or hindering) the understanding of the real potential of the "single pieces" of the entire puzzle.[48]

Another fundamental issue is the one concerning the dosage of cells administered. Attention must be focused on trials using expanded cells, because the number of adipose cells contained in the SVF is obviously limited by the preparation technique as well as by the amount of lipoaspirate that could be reasonably harvested for immediate processing. Conversely, laboratory manipulation of cells allows for a more accurate control of their concentration, with the possibility of having different doses to be tested on patients. Two trials[27,32] looked into this specific issue with contradictory findings: in one trial,[27] only the high-dosage of cells (1×10^8 ASCs) provided significant improvement in clinical scores, radiographic findings, and histologic evaluations compared with the middle and low dosages, whereas in the other study,[32] no correlation between outcome and cell concentration injected was found. Therefore, the question of most appropriate cell concentration/volume remains under debate due to the paucity of data available. Looking at preclinical evidence, it is interesting that in one trial on the rabbit model, it was documented that the best results were obtained with a lower dose of cells (2×10^6), thus suggesting that the complexity of the biological actions of ASCs cannot be explicated just by the "amount effect" related to the number of cells used.[49]

Another interesting issue is related to the harvest site, which is most commonly the abdominal area, followed by buttocks and infrapatellar fat pad. Although harvest from the infrapatellar fat pad allows for a decreased amount of tissue to be harvested compared with the other harvest-site areas, some studies have shown that the "responsiveness" of ASCs from the fat pad is particularly interesting, perhaps related to the fact that infrapatellar fat pad has its own peculiar role in knee anatomy and function.[50] This underscores the theory that even the source of ASCs could be relevant for their biologic properties and their inherent actions. Beyond the aspects related to the product itself, it should be highlighted that the therapeutic effects could be also related to the recipient site, as different joints (ie, shoulder vs knee vs hip) with different biomechanical properties could respond differently to the stimulation provided by ASCs. In the present review, the main focus was knee OA, where ASCs have been tested more extensively compared with other joints. In spite of the fact that we should expect similar outcomes applying ASCs in other joints, as suggested by the few reports already available on hip and ankle application,[20,51] this needs to be confirmed by more robust clinical data.

Notably, OA is often a generic term that actually includes a large spectrum of diseases with different etiopathogenetic pathways, some of which may be more related to inflammation, to mechanical wear (eg, post-meniscectomy OA), or even to genetic predisposition.[52,53] Therefore, the effects of ASC application could change depending on the various etiology of OA.

As should be clear from the present review, many unsolved questions are still pending and, despite an increasing number of in vitro and animal trials, clinical research on ASCs remains in its infancy, and additional clinical data are needed before specific treatments can be recommended.

SUMMARY

The application of ASCs for the treatment of cartilage disease and degeneration represents a fascinating area of research in evolving field of orthobiologics. The abundance of preclinical data suggests that these cells have a number of beneficial actions involving all articular tissues, thus fostering their application in the clinical setting. At the time of publication of this article, the available evidence in knee OA consists of 17 clinical studies, mainly case series with a limited number of patients treated and evaluated at short-term follow-up. Despite these flaws, early clinical results are encouraging, with documented improvement in functional scores and pain relief. When looking at preparation methods, applicative modalities, and formulations, a large variability among studies exists, thus preventing from identifying a best standard of practice. The most commonly adopted strategy consists of the intra-articular injection of the SVF, which is easier to obtain and has lower costs compared with expanded cells, while providing comparable clinical outcomes. In most studies, ASCs were applied together with other biologic agents (such as PRP), therefore hindering the understanding of the real contribution of isolated ASCs to the outcome.

REFERENCES

1. Gomoll AH, Filardo G, de Girolamo L, et al. Surgical treatment for early osteoarthritis. Part I: cartilage repair procedures. Knee Surg Sports Traumatol Arthrosc 2012;20:450–66.
2. Poole AR. What type of cartilage repair are we attempting to attain? J Bone Joint Surg Am 2003;85-A(Suppl):40–4.
3. Kon E, Filardo G, Shani J, et al. Osteochondral regeneration with a novel aragonite-hyaluronate biphasic scaffold: up to 12-month follow-up study in a goat model. J Orthop Surg Res 2015;10:81.
4. Kon E, Filardo G, Perdisa F, et al. Clinical results of multilayered biomaterials for osteochondral regeneration. J Exp Orthop 2014;1:10.
5. Vos T, Flaxman AD, Naghavi M, et al. Years lived with disability (YLDs) for 1160 sequelae of 289 diseases and injuries 1990–2010: a systematic analysis for the Global Burden of Disease Study 2010. Lancet 2012;380: 2163–96.
6. Yoshimura K, Shigeura T, Matsumoto D, et al. Characterization of freshly isolated and cultured cells derived from the fatty and fluid portions of liposuction aspirates. J Cell Physiol 2006;208:64–76.
7. DiMarino AM, Caplan AI, Bonfield TL. Mesenchymal stem cells in tissue repair. Front Immunol 2013;4:201.
8. Caplan AI. Adult mesenchymal stem cells for tissue engineering versus regenerative medicine. J Cell Physiol 2007;213:341–7.
9. Wu L, Cai X, Zhang S, et al. Regeneration of articular cartilage by adipose tissue derived mesenchymal stem cells: perspectives from stem cell biology and molecular medicine. J Cell Physiol 2013;228:938–44.
10. Filardo G, Madry H, Jelic M, et al. Mesenchymal stem cells for the treatment of cartilage lesions: from preclinical findings to clinical application in orthopaedics. Knee Surg Sports Traumatol Arthrosc 2013;21:1717–29.
11. Gimble JM, Katz AJ, Bunnell BA. Adipose-derived stem cells for regenerative medicine. Circ Res 2007;100:1249–60.
12. Zuk PA, Zhu M, Ashjian P, et al. Human adipose tissue is a source of multipotent stem cells. Mol Biol Cell 2002;13:4279–95.
13. Aust L, Devlin B, Foster SJ, et al. Yield of human adipose-derived adult stem cells from liposuction aspirates. Cytotherapy 2004;6:7–14.
14. Oedayrajsingh-Varma MJ, van Ham SM, Knippenberg M, et al. Adipose tissue-derived mesenchymal stem cell yield and growth characteristics are affected by the tissue-harvesting procedure. Cytotherapy 2006;8:166–77.
15. Strioga M, Viswanathan S, Darinskas A, et al. Same or not the same? Comparison of adipose tissue-derived versus bone marrow-derived mesenchymal stem and stromal cells. Stem Cells Dev 2012;21:2724–52.
16. Izadpanah R, Trygg C, Patel B, et al. Biologic properties of mesenchymal stem cells derived from bone marrow and adipose tissue. J Cell Biochem 2006;99: 1285–97.
17. Kern S, Eichler H, Stoeve J, et al. Comparative analysis of mesenchymal stem cells from bone marrow, umbilical cord blood, or adipose tissue. Stem Cells 2006;24:1294–301.

18. De Toni F, Poglio S, Youcef AB, et al. Human adipose-derived stromal cells efficiently support hematopoiesis in vitro and in vivo: a key step for therapeutic studies. Stem Cells Dev 2011;20:2127–38.
19. Somoza RA, Welter JF, Correa D, et al. Chondrogenic differentiation of mesenchymal stem cells: challenges and unfulfilled expectations. Tissue Eng Part B Rev 2014;20:596–608.
20. Pak J. Regeneration of human bones in hip osteonecrosis and human cartilage in knee osteoarthritis with autologous adipose- tissue-derived stem cells: a case series. J Med Case Rep 2011;5:296.
21. Koh YG, Choi YJ. Infrapatellar fat pad-derived mesenchymal stem cell therapy for knee osteoarthritis. Knee 2012;19(6):902–7.
22. Pak J, Chang JJ, Lee JH, et al. Safety reporting on implantation of autologous adipose tissue-derived stem cells with platelet-rich plasma into human articular joints. BMC Musculoskelet Disord 2013;14:337.
23. Pak J, Lee JH, Lee SH. A novel biological approach to treat chondromalacia patellae. PLoS One 2013;8(5):e64569.
24. Koh YG, Choi YJ, Kwon SK, et al. Clinical results and second-look arthroscopic findings after treatment with adipose-derived stem cells for knee osteoarthritis. Knee Surg Sports Traumatol Arthrosc 2015;23(5):1308–16.
25. Koh YG, Jo SB, Kwon OR, et al. Mesenchymal stem cell injections improve symptoms of knee osteoarthritis. Arthroscopy 2013;29(4):748–55.
26. Bui KHT, Duong TD, Nguyen NT, et al. Symptomatic knee osteoarthritis treatment using autologous ASCs and platelet-rich plasma: a clinical study. Biomed Res Ther 2014;1(1):2–8.
27. Jo CH, Lee YG, Shinetal WH. Intra-articular injection of mesenchymal stem cells for the treatment of osteoarthritis of the knee: a proof-of-concept clinical trial. Stem Cells 2014;32(5):1254–66.
28. Koh YG, Choi YJ, Kwon OR, et al. Second-look arthroscopic evaluation of cartilage lesions after mesenchymal stem cell implantation in osteoarthritic knees. Am J Sports Med 2014;42(7):1628–37.
29. Koh YG, Kwon OR, Kim YS, et al. Comparative outcomes of open-wedge high tibial osteotomy with platelet- rich plasma alone or in combination with mesenchymal stem cell treatment: a prospective study. Arthroscopy 2014;30(11):1453–60.
30. Kim YS, Choi YJ, Suh DS, et al. Mesenchymal stem cell implantation in osteoarthritic knees: is fibrin glue effective as a scaffold? Am J Sports Med 2015;43: 176–85.
31. Gibbs N, Diamond R, Sekyere EO, et al. Management of knee osteoarthritis by combined stromal vascular fraction cell therapy, platelet-rich plasma, and musculoskeletal exercises: a case series. J Pain Res 2015;8:799–806.
32. Pers YM, Rackwitz L, Ferreira R, et al. Adipose mesenchymal stromal cell-based therapy for severe osteoarthritis of the knee: a phase I dose-escalation trial. Stem Cells Transl Med 2016;5(7):847–56.
33. Fodor PB, Paulseth SG. Adipose derived stromal cell (ASC) injections for pain management of osteoarthritis in the human knee joint. Aesthet Surg J 2016; 36(2):229–36.
34. Pak J, Lee JH, Park KS, et al. Current use of autologous adipose tissue-derived stromal vascular fraction cells for orthopedic applications. J Biomed Sci 2017; 24(1):9.
35. Spasovski D, Spasovski V, Baščarević Z, et al. Intra-articular injection of autologous adipose-derived mesenchymal stem cells in the treatment of knee osteoarthritis. J Gene Med 2018. [Epub ahead of print].

36. Bansal H, Comella K, Leon J, et al. Intra-articular injection in the knee of adipose derived stromal cells (stromal vascular fraction) and platelet rich plasma for osteoarthritis. J Transl Med 2017;15:141.
37. Mimeault M, Batra SK. Concise review: recent advances on the significance of stem cells in tissue regeneration and cancer therapies. Stem Cells 2006; 24(11):2319–45.
38. González MA, Gonzalez-Rey E, Rico L, et al. Treatment of experimental arthritis by inducing immune tolerance with human adipose-derived mesenchymal stem cells. Arthritis Rheum 2009;60(4):1006–19.
39. Álvaro-Gracia JM, Jover JA, García-Vicuña R, et al. Intravenous administration of expanded allogeneic adipose-derived mesenchymal stem cells in refractory rheumatoid arthritis (Cx611): results of a multicentre, dose escalation, randomised, single-blind, placebo-controlled phase Ib/IIa clinical trial. Ann Rheum Dis 2017;76(1):196–202.
40. ter Huurne M, Schelbergen R, Blattes R, et al. Antiinflammatory and chondroprotective effects of intraarticular injection of adipose-derived stem cells in experimental osteoarthritis. Arthritis Rheum 2012;64(11):3604–13.
41. Mokbel AN, El Tookhy OS, Shamaa AA, et al. Homing and reparative effect of intra-articular injection of autologous mesenchymal stem cells in osteoarthritic animal model. BMC Musculoskelet Disord 2011;12(1):259.
42. Perdisa F, Gostyńska N, Roffi A, et al. Adipose-derived mesenchymal stem cells for the treatment of articular cartilage: a systematic review on preclinical and clinical evidence. Stem Cells Int 2015;2015:597652.
43. Jurgens WJ, Kroeze RJ, Zandieh-Doulabi B, et al. One-step surgical procedure for the treatment of osteochondral defects with adipose-derived stem cells in a caprine knee defect: a pilot study. Biores Open Access 2013; 2(4):315–25.
44. Nam Y, Rim YA, Lee J, et al. Current therapeutic strategies for stem cell-based cartilage regeneration. Stem Cells Int 2018;2018:8490489.
45. Filardo G, Kon E, DI Matteo B, et al. Leukocyte-poor PRP application for the treatment of knee osteoarthritis. Joints 2014;1(3):112–20.
46. Cui L, Wu Y, Cen L, et al. Repair of articular cartilage defect in non-weight bearing areas using ASCs loaded polyglycolic acid mesh. Biomaterials 2009;30(14): 2683–93.
47. Zhang K, Zhang Y, Yan S, et al. Repair of an articular cartilage defect using adipose-derived stem cells loaded on a polyelectrolyte complex scaffold based on poly(l-glutamic acid) and chitosan. Acta Biomater 2013;9(7): 7276–88.
48. Perdisa F, Filardo G, Di Matteo B, et al. Platelet rich plasma: a valid augmentation for cartilage scaffolds? A systematic review. Histol Histopathol 2014; 29(7):805–14.
49. Desando G, Cavallo C, Sartoni F, et al. Intra-articular delivery of adipose derived stromal cells attenuates osteoarthritis progression in an experimental rabbit model. Arthritis Res Ther 2013;15(1):R22.
50. Huri PY, Hamsici S, Ergene E, et al. Infrapatellar fat pad-derived stem cell-based regenerative strategies in orthopedic surgery. Knee Surg Relat Res 2018;30(3): 179–86.
51. Kim YS, Koh YG. Injection of mesenchymal stem cells as a supplementary strategy of marrow stimulation improves cartilage regeneration after lateral sliding calcaneal osteotomy for varus ankle osteoarthritis: clinical and second-look arthroscopic results. Arthroscopy 2016;32(5):878–89.

52. Aigner T, Fundel K, Saas J, et al. Large-scale gene expression profiling reveals major pathogenetic pathways of cartilage degeneration in osteoarthritis. Arthritis Rheum 2006;54(11):3533–44.
53. Selmi C, Kon E, De Santis M, et al. How advances in personalized medicine will change rheumatology. Per Med 2018;15(2):75–8.

Orthobiologics for Bone Healing

Jacob G. Calcei, MD*, Scott A. Rodeo, MD

KEYWORDS

- Orthobiologics • Bone healing • Fracture healing • Tendon-to-bone • Bone grafting
- Nonunion

KEY POINTS

- Orthobiologics are a group of biological materials and substrates that promote bone, ligament, muscle, and tendon healing.
- Orthobiologics in bone healing and tendon-to-bone healing include bone grafts, bone graft substitutes, growth factors, cell-signaling proteins, and cell-based therapies.
- Properties of orthobiologics in bone healing include osteoconduction, osteoinduction, and osteogenesis.
- Further investigation of orthobiologics with high-quality clinical trials is needed.

INTRODUCTION

In all subspecialties of orthopedic surgery, bone healing is an important process that must be appreciated and understood. Specifically, in sports medicine orthopedic surgery, bone healing comes into play in several scenarios from the more common challenges of fracture healing or anterior cruciate ligament (ACL) bone-tendon-bone incorporation to relatively uncommon cases such as bony avulsion healing or bone grafting tunnels in revision ACL reconstruction. A sports medicine surgeon must have a diverse toolbox in order to address these often complex cases, and orthobiologics are a growing part of that expanding toolbox.

Orthobiologics are a group of biological materials and substrates including bone grafts, bone graft substitutes, growth factors, cell-signaling proteins, and cell-based therapies that promote bone, ligament, muscle, and tendon healing. Properties of orthobiologics in bone healing, including osteoconduction, osteoinduction, and osteogenesis, are part of the "diamond concept" of fracture healing described by Giannoudis and colleagues,[1] which includes osteogenic cells, osteoconductive

---

Disclosure Statement: The authors have no conflicts or funding sources related to this article.
a Department of Sports Medicine and Shoulder, Hospital for Special Surgery, 535 E 70th Street, New York, NY 10021, USA
* Corresponding author.
E-mail address: calceij@hss.edu

scaffolds, osteoinductive growth factors, and mechanical stability. This article discusses the important properties of orthobiologics in bone healing, many of the orthobiologics currently available for bone healing, the related literature, their current clinical uses in sports medicine, and systemic factors that inhibit bone healing.

OSTEOCONDUCTION, OSTEOINDUCTION, AND OSTEOGENESIS

Osteoconduction, osteoinduction, and osteogenesis are the 3 major properties of orthobiologics used in bone healing. The ability of specific orthobiologics to successfully aid in bone healing is determined by these 3 properties.[2] Depending on the problem at hand and the intended use of the orthobiologic material, these properties determine which substance is most appropriate, and this specific material is often affected by cost and access to each material, as well as the associated comorbidities and contraindications. The basic osteoconductive, osteoinductive, and osteogenic potential of various currently available agents are outlined later in this article (**Table 1**).

Osteoconduction is a bone formation process where an ingrowth of the host cells, tissues, and vasculature occurs passively, aided by an introduced scaffold.[3-5] Therefore, osteoconductive materials serve as a scaffold for the host response to use in order to heal or form new bone. Examples of osteoconductive materials are bone autograft, bone allograft, demineralized bone matrix (DBM), and inert filler structures such as calcium ceramics. Osteoconductive materials often contain a similar structured matrix to that of cancellous bone in order to support the ingrowth of host cells and vasculature. Cancellous autograft, therefore, has the greatest osteoconductive potential compared with growth factors and signaling molecules such as bone morphogenetic proteins (BMPs), which have no specific physical scaffold structure when used alone.[5]

Osteoinduction is a bone formation process where new bone is generated and supported by specific growth factors from the introduced substance that promote differentiation of mesenchymal stem cells to osteoblasts and chondroblasts. Examples of osteoinductive orthobiologics primarily include growth factors and signaling

Table 1
Orthobiologics and their specific osteoconductive, osteoinductive, and osteogenic properties

	Osteoconductive	Osteoinductive	Osteogenic
Cortical autograft	+	+	+
Cancellous autograft	+++	+++	+++
Cortical allograft	+	+/-	-
Cancellous allograft	+	+/-	-
Demineralized bone matrix	+	++	-
Calcium ceramics	+	-	-
Bone marrow aspirate	-	++	+++
Bone morphogenetic protein	-	++	-
Platelet-rich plasma	-	+++	+

+, activity; -, no activity; +/-, activity depends on preparation process.
Adapted from Bray CC, Walker CM, Spence DD. Orthobiologics in pediatric sports medicine. Orthop Clin North Am 2017;48(3):334; with permission.

molecules such as BMPs, platelet-derived growth factor (PDGF), fibroblast growth factor, and interleukins, among others, as well as bone autograft, bone marrow aspirate concentrate (BMAC), and platelet-rich plasma (PRP).[3–5]

Osteogenesis is the process by which specific cellular elements within the graft are able to synthesize new bone. Autogenous cancellous bone has excellent osteogenic potential, because it has all of the necessary elements to stimulate osteogenesis; however, as our understanding of the cellular and molecular mechanisms involved in bone healing expands, additional orthobiologics have emerged, including growth factors, cell signaling proteins, and cell-based therapies.

ORTHOBIOLOGICS IN BONE HEALING

This article discusses the various orthobiologics in sports medicine, including bone graft options, cell-based therapies, and growth factors, as well as the current supporting literature for each substance.

Bone Grafts

Autologous bone grafts

Autologous bone grafts contain all 3 important properties to promote bone healing: osteoconduction, osteoinduction, and osteogenesis. The use of bone autograft to supplement bone healing has an extensive history in orthopedic surgery and has long been considered the "gold standard" for augmentation of bone healing in the treatment of delayed unions and nonunions.[2,6,7] Autologous bone grafts come in a few forms, including cancellous, vascularized cortical, and nonvascularized cortical. Cancellous bone autograft has the greatest osteoconductive, osteoinductive, and osteogenic potential of the 3; however cancellous autograft does not provide immediate structural support.[4] Therefore, if the intended function of the graft is to serve as a structural support, a cortical graft is preferred, and given the morbidity associated with obtaining cortical autograft, structural cortical allograft is often preferred.[4,8]

Autologous iliac crest bone graft (ICBG) remains the gold standard because it contains the structure of cortical bone combined with the bone healing properties of cancellous bone autograft.[7] However, the potential morbidity associated with traditional techniques for harvesting autologous ICBG has led to the development of alternative methods to harvest bone autograft, such as reamer-irrigator-aspirator.[9] Regardless of the method used to obtain the autologous bone graft or the chosen site to harvest the graft, bone autograft remains a powerful tool in bone healing, especially in the setting of nonunion and revision surgeries where bone healing is required over bone void filling.[3]

Bone allograft and demineralized bone matrix

Allografts are typically used as space fillers and structural struts. The osteoconductive properties of cancellous bone allograft allow it to be incorporated into the host bone and serves as a void filler, whereas the structural properties of cortical allograft allow it to be used in cases where physical support is necessary, such as elevating the articular surface in a tibial plateau fracture. Morselized and cancellous allografts are freeze-dried cancellous bone chips with similar osteoconductive properties to cancellous autograft and are typically used to fill bone defects such as those created by cyst curettage or occurring in the setting of a large depressed articular fracture. These allograft cancellous chips have similar biomechanical properties to that of metaphyseal bone in that they can provide some mechanical support in compression.[4] Cortical and osteochondral allografts are more structurally sound and are typically used as cortical struts in trauma or for limb salvage procedures in oncology. The use of cortical and osteochondral allografts in sports medicine is seen in procedures such as realignment osteotomies for malalignment (ie, high tibial osteotomy, distal femoral osteotomy), mosaicplasty for large osteochondral defects, or bone/joint augmentation in the case of glenoid reconstruction.

DBM is an osteoconductive and osteoinductive bone graft substitute, which is composed of bone allograft with inorganic materials removed. The osteoinductive potential of DBM comes from the measurable amounts of BMP and vascular endothelial growth factor (VEGF).[6] Initial studies in animals and humans demonstrated efficacy of DBM in comparison to open autologous grafting in fracture care more than 20 years ago.[10,11] These findings were further supported more recently by Desai and colleagues,[12] where they suggested that DBM may be superior to BMP-2 when used in conjunction with BMAC in healing tibial nonunions. In addition, Lareau and colleagues[13] presented a series of 25 fifth metatarsal Jones fractures in National Football League players, most treated with screw fixation supplemented with BMAC and DBM, with a 100% rate of return to play with an in-season average return to play of 8.7 weeks.

Bone graft substitutes

Synthetic calcium salt–based substitutes that have been manufactured to mimic the osteoconductive properties of bone graft include calcium sulfate, calcium phosphate, tricalcium phosphate, and coralline hydroxyapatite. These osteoconductive alternatives are often used as void fillers in larger segmental defects or, in the case of infection, can be mixed with antibiotics. Moreover, these synthetics may be combined with biologically active osteoinductive and osteogenic substrates such as BMAC, PRP, or BMPs. There are various options for synthetic bone graft substitute, all of which have a similar compressive strength to that of cancellous bone, with the exception of calcium phosphate, which has a compressive strength up to 10 times that of cancellous bone and has a slower resorption rate compared with other synthetics.[5]

Cell Therapies

Bone marrow aspirate concentrate

Autologous bone marrow aspirate has demonstrated positive outcomes in the treatment of various musculoskeletal injuries—bone and soft tissue alike. Bone marrow, specifically red marrow, contains 2 types of adult stem cells: hematopoietic stem cells and mesenchymal stem cells (MSCs).[14] The minimum criteria to define human MSCs as set forth by the Mesenchymal and Tissue Stem Cell Committee of the International Society for Cellular Therapy are the following: (1) MSCs must be plastic-adherent when maintained in standard culture conditions; (2) MSCs must express CD105, CD73, and CD90 and lack expression of CD45, CD34, CD14, or CD11b, CD79alpha, or CD19, and HLA-DR surface molecules; and (3) MSCs must differentiate to osteoblasts, adipocytes, and chondroblasts in vitro.[15] Given the bone-forming potential of MSCs, BMAC, which has been proposed as a means of concentrating MSCs, has garnered the attention of surgeons treating patients with fractures, fusions, and just about any other musculoskeletal issue (**Fig. 1**). The ultimate goal of BMAC in bone healing is to maximize the number of progenitor cells delivered in the aspirate. Hernigou and colleagues[16] reported that concentrated bone marrow aspirate had an average of more than 2500 progenitor cells/cm³, whereas aspirate before concentration had just more than 600 progenitor cells/cm³. The underlying biological mechanism supporting the use of BMAC in bone healing is related to the ability of MSCs to differentiate into osteoprogenitor cells that then differentiate into osteoblasts when surrounded by the proper growth factors and cytokines.[17,18] Additional mechanisms for the positive effect of BMAC include a paracrine action whereby cytokines

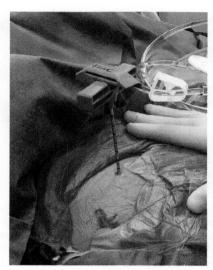

Fig. 1. Iliac crest aspiration prep and needle using the bone marrow aspirate concentrate system (Bone Marrow Aspirate Concentrate (BMAC®) System, Harvest Terumo BCT, Lakewood, CO, USA). The aspiration trochar is inserted into the iliac wing and advanced between the inner and outer tables of the iliac crest. (*Courtesy of* Harvest Terumo BCT, Inc, Lakewood, CO; with permission.)

produced by the marrow cells stimulate endogenous local and possibly distant host cells and the presence of endothelial progenitor cells in BMAC that induce angiogenesis and restore blood flow to the fracture site.[5]

Animal studies examining the impact of BMAC on bone healing have demonstrated significantly more bone formation in fractures treated with BMAC. Gianakos and colleagues[19] reviewed the results of 35 studies where long bone defects in animals were treated with BMAC and found that 100% showed increased osteogenesis and 90% demonstrated significantly more bone formation compared with controls based on histologic analysis. Clinical outcomes studies have demonstrated similar results. Hernigou and colleagues[16,20] described harvest of bone marrow aspirate from the iliac crest, concentration via centrifugation, and percutaneous injection into the fracture site in 60 atrophic tibial shaft nonunions, with union achieved in 53 of the patients. They found that the number of progenitor cells measured in the grafting material was significantly higher in the patients who achieved successful union. Because BMAC is a liquid and therefore can seep away from the fracture site, it is often combined with an osteoconductive scaffold, such as DBM, allograft, or ceramic grafts to serve as a carrier vehicle and to provide structural support (**Fig. 2**).[3,5] A cohort study by Desai and colleagues,[12] using a combination of BMAC and DBM for percutaneous treatment of atrophic tibial nonunion, attained a rate of healing of 86% at 4.5 months. Overall, the use of BMAC in bone healing has demonstrated positive results and continues to be used in the treatment of atrophic nonunions. Although the indications for the use of BMAC in the treatment of acute fractures are not as well established, Schottel and Warner describe their indications for supplementing primary fracture fixation with allograft and BMAC.[18]

Platelet-rich plasma

PRP has been a particular focus of recent research. PRP is prepared from an autologous suspension of platelets extracted from the patient's whole blood via centrifugation techniques (**Fig. 3**).[3,5] Platelets have demonstrated osteoinductive properties

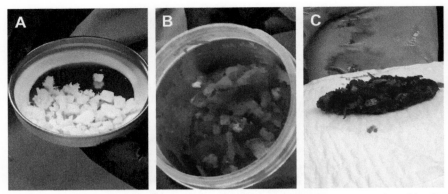

Fig. 2. BMAC is mixed with allograft cancellous chips and DBM for ACL tunnel grafting in a 2-stage revision ACL reconstruction. (*A*) Allograft cancellous bone chips. (*B*) BMAC mixed with allograft cancellous chips and DBM (Grafton DBM, BioHorizons, Birmingham, AL, USA). (*C*) Mixture of BMAC, allograft chips, and DBM formed to be inserted into the bone void of primary ACL tunnels.

because they are rich in important growth factors. Specifically, the alpha granules in platelets contain and release numerous growth factors, including PDGF, transforming growth factor β1 (TGF-β1), VEGF, epidermal growth factor, fibroblast growth factor, and insulin-like growth factor 1.[3] The widespread use of PRP in orthopedics extends to bone healing, where PRP has shown positive results. For example, PRP injected into the fracture site of a long bone atrophic nonunion resulted in 87% (82/94) union at 4 months.[21] A comparison of PRP with exchange intramedullary nailing for long bone nonunions resulted in a healing rate of approximately 93% in the PRP group compared with 80% in the exchange nailing group.[22] These studies point toward the promising potential of PRP in fracture healing, although further investigation is needed. In ACL reconstruction, although PRP supplementation has provided some preliminary evidence of accelerated graft maturation, studies have yet to demonstrate an improvement in tendon-to-bone healing.[23–25]

Despite the widespread use of PRP for the treatment of various musculoskeletal issues, the exact biological composition and its effects on musculoskeletal healing

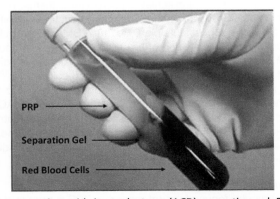

PRP

Separation Gel

Red Blood Cells

Fig. 3. PRP using a separation acid citrate dextrose (ACD) separation gel. Red blood cells are concentrated at the bottom of the test tube, whereas the PRP is above the separation gel at the top of the tube.

remains unclear. One of the major issues with PRP is that there are numerous prepa- ration protocols, all resulting in a different product that is injected back into the patient. A systematic review of 105 studies revealed that only 16% reliably reported quantita- tive PRP composition and only 10% clearly reported the preparation protocol.[26] This study points to the need for identification of sentinel markers to characterize PRP and standardized assays and methods in order to quantify the composition and biological activity. A more detailed analysis beyond simple measures such as platelet or white blood cell count is required to be able to predict biological activity of PRP formula- tions.[27] Murray and colleagues[28] described a 23-item checklist for the minimum reporting requirements for studies evaluating PRP based on expert consensus, which aims to improve the quality and reproducibility of PRP-related research.

Osteoinductive Growth Factors and Proteins

Bone morphogenetic protein

BMPs are members of the TGF-β superfamily and contain osteoinductive and osteo- genic properties. BMPs play a role in osteoblast differentiation, osteogenesis, and angio- genesis through their function in complex signaling pathways.[5] BMPs require a carrier vehicle, such as collagen sponges and calcium ceramics, to deliver and maintain the liquid BMP near the fracture site.[5] BMP-2 and BMP-7 have been approved by the US Food and Drug Administration (FDA) for use in long bone nonunions, open tibia fractures, and spinal fusion.[6,29] Current off-label use includes foot and ankle arthrodesis proced- ures, treatment of high-risk fractures, and nonunions.[30] The 2 commercially available re- combinant human BMPs (rhBMPs) approved for clinical use are INFUSE (Medtronic Sofamor Danek, Memphis, TN, USA), rhBMP-2 and OP-1 Putty (Stryker Biotech, Hop- kinton, MA, USA), rhBMP-7.[31] Despite the literature supporting the powerful inductive potential of BMPs, their use in fracture healing has fallen out of favor in comparison with the other orthobiologics. This is because they are expensive and there are several morbidities associated with its use, including excess heterotopic bone formation (espe- cially given the tendency of liquid BMP to seep into the surrounding soft tissue), the remote potential for carcinogenesis, renal and hepatic failure, and compartment syn- drome.[3,5,32] At this time, the indications for the use of BMP in sports medicine outside of the treatment of atrophic nonunions are unclear and warrant further investigation.

Platelet-derived growth factor

PDGF is a signaling molecule that is released by degranulating platelets in the early phases of fracture healing through its important role in chemotaxis.[33,34] In bone heal- ing, recombinant human PDGF (rhPDGF) has been approved by the FDA for hindfoot ankle fusions. A randomized controlled trial of 434 patients undergoing hindfoot or ankle arthrodesis reported no difference in fusion rate between the group augmented with autograft and the group augmented with beta-tricalcium phosphate osteocon- ductive matrix plus rhPDGF-BB homodimer, which is a specific PDGF isoform found in bone (Augment Bone Graft; Wright Medical Group Inc., Memphis, TN, USA).[35] An animal study by Bordei examining the effects of locally applied PDGF on tibia fracture healing in rats demonstrated improved fracture callus consolidation at all time points (3, 7, and 10 days) in the PDGF-treated group compared with the control group.[36]

In humans, a recent prospective randomized pilot study examined the effects of rhPDGF-BB (Augment Bone Graft; Wright Medical Group Inc., Memphis, TN, USA) on healing in human distal radius fractures and found rhPDGF-BB to be safe with no adverse events recorded, although there was also no improvement in fracture healing between the rhPDGF-BB and control groups.[37] Thus, local use of PDGF in fracture healing seems safe and may have positive clinical implications, although future larger-scale clinical trials are needed. Currently, there are no PDGF agents approved specifically for use in fracture healing. PDGF has demonstrated promising results in tendon-to-bone healing in animal studies. Tokunaga and colleagues[38] found significantly improved collagen fiber orientation, stiffness, stress to failure, and ultimate load to failure with a PDGF-BB gel compared with a control in healing of rotator cuff tendon-to-bone in rats.

Parathyroid hormone

Calcium and phosphate metabolism are regulated in part by parathyroid hormone (PTH). Recombinant human PTH (rhPTH), in the form of teriparatide, is the only anabolic agent that is FDA-approved for use in osteoporosis because its use is associated with an increase in bone mineral density and decreased fracture risk.[39,40] The use of rhPTH in sports medicine has been examined in fracture healing and tendon-to-bone healing in animal models.

Animal studies have demonstrated positive effects of rhPTH on fracture healing with improved bone mineral density and callus formation, accelerated healing and formation of lamellar bone, and increased strength.[41–44] A recent animal study by Zhang and colleagues[45] demonstrated a similar improvement in fracture healing, bone mass, and bone microarchitecture with less frequent, once-weekly dosing of rhPTH. These animal-study results have translated to early human studies. In a randomized controlled trial of 102 postmenopausal women with distal radius fractures treated with closed reduction supplemented with PTH versus placebo, Aspenberg and colleagues[46] found a significantly shorter time to fracture healing in patients treated with daily injections of 20 μg rhPTH compared with placebo. In a randomized, placebo-controlled pilot study, Almirol and colleagues[47] showed significantly increased bone formation biomarkers N-terminal propeptide of type 1 procollagen and osteocalcin in premenopausal women with lower extremity stress fractures treated with 20 μg rhPTH daily compared with placebo. Currently, there are several ongoing clinical trials examining the effects of rhPTH on fracture healing in humans, which will help clarify the role of rhPTH in fracture healing. In the sports medicine arena, rhPTH may have efficacy for stress fractures.

In an animal study examining the effect of rhPTH on tendon-to-bone healing, Hettrich and colleagues[48] found histologic evidence of more fibrocartilage, osteoblasts, and angiogenesis in rats treated with rhPTH after an induced supraspinatus tear and repair compared with controls. Collagen fiber orientation was also significantly improved in the treatment group at the later time points. The reported histologic improvements, however, did not result in improved biomechanical properties.

Vitamin D and calcium

Vitamin D is a well-established factor in bone health and an essential player in bone mineralization. Therefore, vitamin D plays a role in bone healing through callous formation and bone remodeling. A systematic review examining the role that vitamin D plays in fracture healing found variable results in preclinical studies investigating the effect of vitamin D on the specific stages of bone healing.[49] Vitamin D supplementation has been shown to stimulate osteoblastogenesis,[50] increase the production of osteocalcin and osteopontin,[51] and stimulate osteoclast-mediated bone resorption,[52] among many other biological functions.[49] Clinical studies have shown calcium and vitamin D supplementation to significantly increase bone mineral density and callus area in proximal humerus and distal radius fracture patients, respectively.[53,54] Much of the literature on vitamin D plus calcium supplementation has focused on fracture prevention, where a Cochran review found a slight benefit in the prevention of fractures, especially hip fractures, with calcium and vitamin D supplementation, but no significant benefit with vitamin D supplementation alone.[55] Low vitamin D levels have resulted in decreased bone formation and less collagen fiber organization in a rat rotator cuff repair model.[56] It is clear that vitamin D plays a role in bone and tendon healing, but the specific biological mechanisms involved remain unclear.

APPLICATIONS OF ORTHOBIOLOGICS
Orthobiologics in Delayed Union and Nonunion

In the case of fracture healing, a combination of biomechanical stability and favorable biology determine whether a fracture will go on to a successful union. When union is delayed or has failed, orthobiologics may be used to supplement fixation and lead to effective bone healing. Delayed union is defined as a fracture that remains unhealed after 4 months. The FDA defines a fracture nonunion as a fracture that is 9 months old, with no signs of healing for 3 months,[5] whereas others define a fracture as a nonunion when bone healing has not been achieved by 6 months.[57,58] Nonunion can be further divided into 2 categories: hypertrophic and atrophic. Hypertrophic nonunion typically forms in a setting where the biology is favorable, but the skeletal fixation method is mechanically insufficient, resulting in motion at the fracture site with resultant callus formation but failed union. Conversely, atrophic nonunions have minimal callus formation and are the result of poor biological conditions at the fracture site, such as inadequate vascularity or metabolic conditions.[5,57] Treatment of hypertrophic nonunions aims to decrease motion at the fracture site by improving the mechanical skeletal fixation, whereas treatment for atrophic nonunions aims at improving the biological environment at the fracture site. Depending on the baseline comorbidities of the patient, orthobiologics and cell therapies may be used from the onset at the time of initial fixation to maximize biological potential and avoid delayed union or nonunion.

Orthobiologics are often used to augment fixation and improve the biology for bone healing, especially in the case of atrophic nonunion. Autologous bone graft remains the gold standard because it possesses all 3 important properties that promote bone healing—osteoconduction, osteoinduction, and osteogenesis—although it is associated with the comorbidities related to obtaining the graft. As mentioned earlier, the use of BMAC plus DBM has demonstrated excellent results in the treatment of atrophic nonunion. Hernigou and colleagues[16] demonstrated an 88% (53/60) healing rate in atrophic nonunions treated with percutaneous injection of BMAC alone, whereas Desai and colleagues[12] used a combination of DBM plus BMAC for a healing rate of 86% at 4.5 months in tibial atrophic nonunions. rhBMP-2 in combination with allograft cancellous chips has exhibited comparable results to autograft alone in the treatment of tibial shaft fractures with extensive bone loss.[59] Findings by Giannoudis and colleagues[60] in the treatment of nonunion suggest that rhBMP-7 has a synergistic effect when combined with autograft because they achieved 100% union in their series of 45 patients with aseptic atrophic nonunions. PRP alone has also demonstrated good potential in treating fracture nonunions, with reported union rates of 87% and 93% in 2 studies.[21,22] Therefore, although nonunions remain a difficult problem, the emergence of orthobiologics, especially in the case of atrophic nonunion, has given orthopedic surgeons several effective tools.

Tendon-To-Bone Healing

Successful ACL reconstruction begins with proper graft choice and tunnel placement, but the biology of tendon-to-bone healing in order to promote graft incorporation and bone ingrowth has a large impact on the long-term success of the ligament reconstruction.[61] The initial step in tendon-to-bone healing is the formation of a fibrovascular granulation tissue connecting the tendon and bone, which is followed by bone ingrowth and an eventual reformation of the collagen fiber structure at the tendon-bone interface.[62] Animal studies have demonstrated that local delivery of rhBMP-2 accelerates bone ingrowth, improves osteointegration, and increases stiffness in tendon graft incorporation into a bone tunnel.[63,64] The use of MSCs to improve tendon-to-bone healing has been investigated in animal studies. Lui and colleagues[65] reported improved early ACL graft-healing in a rat model with ACL grafts wrapped in a tendon-derived stem cell sheet. Preclinical studies examining the role of MMPs in graft healing have demonstrated improved tendon graft-to-bone tunnel healing with MMP inhibition, which may have a positive effect via inhibition of bone resorption at the healing interface.[66]

Animal models for rotator cuff tendon-to-bone healing have shown promising results. Rodeo and colleagues[67] reported significantly greater failure loads at 6 and 12 weeks in a sheep rotator cuff repair model with an osteoinductive growth factor mixture. Improved collagen fiber orientation, stiffness, stress to failure, and ultimate load to failure was found in a rat rotator cuff model with a PDGF-BB gel compared with controls in a rat model of rotator cuff tendon-to-bone healing.[38] However, although Kovacevic and colleagues[68] found increased angiogenesis and cellular proliferation in rat rotator cuff repairs with rhPDGF-BB, strength of the repair was not increased. The introduction of a calcium phosphate matrix at the tendon-bone interface has demonstrated an improved tendon-to-bone healing in a rat model in multiple studies.[69,70] These studies, among others, reveal the potential for orthobiologics to improve tendon-to-bone healing.

Revision Anterior Cruciate Ligament Reconstruction and Tunnel Grafting

Bone resorption and tunnel widening after ACL reconstruction is a well-recognized phenomenon.[61,71] In the case of a failed ACL reconstruction requiring revision, large bone tunnel defects can pose a challenge and often require bone grafting as part of a single- or 2-stage procedure (**Fig. 4**). Although there is no clear consensus, bone tunnel grafting is recommended when the bone tunnel widening is greater than 12 to 15 mm, when there is tunnel malpositioning, or if the proposed revised tunnels are within the border of the primary tunnels.[72,73] Several approaches using various bone grafts and single-stage versus two-stage techniques have been described including single-stage allograft dowels,[74] single-stage calcium phosphate bone cement,[75] 2-stage allograft bone matrix,[76] and 2-stage allograft dowels,[77] among others. Yamaguchi and colleagues[78] describe their technique for a 2-stage bone-grafting approach for revision ACL reconstruction, which includes arthroscopic delivery of a bone allograft matrix composed of 5 mL Stimublast DBM Putty (Arthrex, Naples, FL, USA) and 5 mL FlexiGRAFT cortical fibers (Arthrex, Naples, FL, USA), mixed with PRP per tunnel. The optimal strategy for bone grafting in a single- or 2-staged fashion remains unclear.

Orthobiologics and Osteotomies

An area of sports medicine where orthobiologics are frequently used for bone healing is limb realignment via osteotomy. A systematic review examined the use of various bone void fillers for opening-wedge osteotomies in the knee.[79] Autograft was used in 29.5% of cases, allograft in 25.9%, and no filler was used in 17.3% of cases. The investigators found significantly lower rates of delayed and nonunion with autograft compared with allograft, whereas both autograft and allograft had lower rates of delayed/nonunion compared with synthetic bone graft substitutes.

Giuseffi and colleagues[80] presented a review of 100 opening-wedge high tibial osteotomies treated with plate fixation and bone grafting. Nonunion was associated

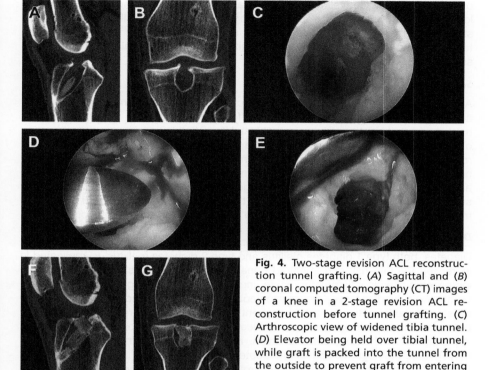

Fig. 4. Two-stage revision ACL reconstruction tunnel grafting. (*A*) Sagittal and (*B*) coronal computed tomography (CT) images of a knee in a 2-stage revision ACL reconstruction before tunnel grafting. (*C*) Arthroscopic view of widened tibia tunnel. (*D*) Elevator being held over tibial tunnel, while graft is packed into the tunnel from the outside to prevent graft from entering the joint. (*E*) Arthroscopic view of tibial tunnel packed with bone marrow aspirate concentrate mixed with allograft cancellous chips and DBM. (*F*) Sagittal and (*G*) coronal CT images after tunnel grafting.

with allograft plus DBM, whereas there were no cases of nonunion in patients treated with allograft plus bone marrow aspirate or iliac crest bone autograft. A recent study examining the 5-year survivorship in lateral opening-wedge distal femoral osteotomies for valgus deformity demonstrated 74% survivorship in the group treated for isolated lateral compartment arthritis and 92% survivorship in the group that underwent a concomitant joint preservation procedure. The osteotomy was fixed with a lateral locking plate, with most supplemented with iliac crest autograft and allograft cancellous chips, and there was only 1 nonunion after a failure of the medial bone hinge.[81]

SYSTEMIC INHIBITORY FACTORS
Nonsteroidal Antiinflammatory Drugs

Nonsteroidal antiinflammatory drugs (NSAIDs) are widely used in sports medicine and have been linked to decreased bone healing. NSAIDs work by inhibiting COX-2 and therefore decrease prostaglandin production, which are an important part of the inflammatory process in the acute phase of bone healing.[31] High doses of NSAIDs have resulted in impaired fracture healing in animal studies and have the biggest impact in the acute inflammatory stage.[82] Clinical studies have shown high local concentrations of NSAIDs to be associated with delayed union and nonunion.[83] A recent animal study demonstrated impaired tendon-to-bone healing in the presence of a COX-2 inhibitor in a rabbit ACL model.[84] Despite these findings, a systematic review of the quality of studies related to NSAIDs and bone healing found poorer methodologic quality in studies that reported a negative effect of NSAIDs compared with studies reporting that NSAIDs are safe for use in bone healing.[85] This study points to the need for quality prospective randomized controlled clinical trials to clarify the safety of NSAID use in bone healing.

Smoking

Among the myriad of negative health effects associated with smoking, it is widely accepted that smoking has an adverse effect on bone healing. Preclinical studies have shown that nicotine reduces osteoblast differentiation and decreases proliferation of human MSCs.[86,87] Nicotine also caused a delay in tendon-to-bone healing in a rat rotator cuff repair model.[88] Clinical studies have shown longer time to union and higher nonunion rates, as well as a trend toward increased postoperative rates of superficial and deep infection after surgical management in smokers compared with nonsmokers.[89–92] In addition, studies suggest that smoking cessation, even if temporary, may lead to improved bone and soft-tissue healing with fewer complications.[93]

Diabetes

Diabetes, both type 1 diabetes mellitus and type 2 diabetes mellitus, is implicated in increased fracture risk and impaired bone healing. Diabetes is associated with an increased systemic inflammatory state, increased reactive oxygen species, and hyperglycemia, leading to a decrease in osteoblast number and function and an increase in osteoclast differentiation and subsequent bone resorption.[94] Fracture healing in diabetic patients is prolonged with a significantly higher risk of complications such as impaired wound healing, delayed union, and nonunion.[94–96] Insulin administration may reverse the negative effects of diabetes on bone healing.[94] In a rat model of rotator cuff tendon repair, sustained hyperglycemia impaired tendon-to-bone healing based on histologic and biomechanical criteria.[97]

SUMMARY

The emergence of orthobiologics and the new frontier of growth factor and cell-based therapies have expanded the orthopedic surgeon's toolbox, especially for bone healing. Orthobiologics beyond bone grafts and bone graft substitutes, including growth factors, proteins, and cell-based therapies, have demonstrated an ability to promote successful bone healing, even in difficult situations. Although further investigation with high-quality clinical trials is needed before many of these treatments become standard of care, the future is bright for orthobiologics in bone healing.

REFERENCES

1. Giannoudis PV, Einhorn TA, Marsh D. Fracture healing: the diamond concept. Injury 2007;38(Suppl 4):S3–6.
2. Egol KA, Nauth A, Lee M, et al. Bone grafting: sourcing, timing, strategies, and alternatives. J Orthop Trauma 2015;29(Suppl 12):S10–4.
3. Bray CC, Walker CM, Spence DD. Orthobiologics in pediatric sports medicine. Orthop Clin North Am 2017;48(3):333–42.
4. Finkemeier CG. Bone-grafting and bone-graft substitutes. J Bone Joint Surg Am 2002;84-A(3):454–64.
5. Roberts TT, Rosenbaum AJ. Bone grafts, bone substitutes and orthobiologics: the bridge between basic science and clinical advancements in fracture healing. Organogenesis 2012;8(4):114–24.

6. Nauth A, Lane J, Watson JT, et al. Bone graft substitution and augmentation. J Orthop Trauma 2015;29(Suppl 12):S34–8.

7. Sen MK, Miclau T. Autologous iliac crest bone graft: should it still be the gold standard for treating nonunions? Injury 2007;38(Suppl 1):S75–80.

8. Berkes MB, Little MT, Schottel PC, et al. Outcomes of Schatzker II tibial plateau fracture open reduction internal fixation using structural bone allograft. J Orthop Trauma 2014;28(2):97–102.

9. Sagi HC, Young ML, Gerstenfeld L, et al. Qualitative and quantitative differences between bone graft obtained from the medullary canal (with a Reamer/Irrigator/Aspirator) and the iliac crest of the same patient. J Bone Joint Surg Am 2012; 94(23):2128–35.

10. Tiedeman JJ, Connolly JF, Strates BS, et al. Treatment of nonunion by percutaneous injection of bone marrow and demineralized bone matrix. An experimental study in dogs. Clin Orthop Relat Res 1991;268:294–302.

11. Tiedeman JJ, Garvin KL, Kile TA, et al. The role of a composite, demineralized bone matrix and bone marrow in the treatment of osseous defects. Orthopedics 1995;18(12):1153–8.

12. Desai P, Hasan SM, Zambrana L, et al. Bone mesenchymal stem cells with growth factors successfully treat nonunions and delayed unions. HSS J 2015;11(2):104–11.

13. Lareau CR, Hsu AR, Anderson RB. Return to play in national football league players after operative jones fracture treatment. Foot Ankle Int 2016;37(1):8–16.

14. Hernigou P, Poignard A, Manicom O, et al. The use of percutaneous autologous bone marrow transplantation in nonunion and avascular necrosis of bone. J Bone Joint Surg Br 2005;87(7):896–902.

15. Dominici M, Le Blanc K, Mueller I, et al. Minimal criteria for defining multipotent mesenchymal stromal cells. The International Society for Cellular Therapy position statement. Cytotherapy 2006;8(4):315–7.

16. Hernigou P, Poignard A, Beaujean F, et al. Percutaneous autologous bone-marrow grafting for nonunions. Influence of the number and concentration of progenitor cells. J Bone Joint Surg Am 2005;87(7):1430–7.

17. Crane JL, Cao X. Bone marrow mesenchymal stem cells and TGF-β signaling in bone remodeling. J Clin Invest 2014;124(2):466–72.

18. Schottel PC, Warner SJ. Role of bone marrow aspirate in orthopedic trauma. Orthop Clin North Am 2017;48(3):311–21.

19. Gianakos A, Ni A, Zambrana L, et al. Bone marrow aspirate concentrate in animal long bone healing: an analysis of basic science evidence. J Orthop Trauma 2016; 30(1):1–9.

20. Hernigou P, Mathieu G, Poignard A, et al. Percutaneous autologous bone-marrow grafting for nonunions. Surgical technique. J Bone Joint Surg Am 2006;88(Suppl 1 Pt 2):322–7.

21. Malhotra R, Kumar V, Garg B, et al. Role of autologous platelet-rich plasma in treatment of long-bone nonunions: a prospective study. Musculoskelet Surg 2015;99(3):243–8.

22. Duramaz A, Ursavaş HT, Bilgili MG, et al. Platelet-rich plasma versus exchange intramedullary nailing in treatment of long bone oligotrophic nonunions. Eur J Orthop Surg Traumatol 2018;28(1):131–7.

23. Hutchinson ID, Rodeo SA, Perrone GS, et al. Can platelet-rich plasma enhance anterior cruciate ligament and meniscal repair? J Knee Surg 2015;28(1):19–28.

24. Orrego M, Larrain C, Rosales J, et al. Effects of platelet concentrate and a bone plug on the healing of hamstring tendons in a bone tunnel. Arthroscopy 2008; 24(12):1373–80.

25. Radice F, Yánez R, Gutiérrez V, et al. Comparison of magnetic resonance imaging findings in anterior cruciate ligament grafts with and without autologous platelet-derived growth factors. Arthroscopy 2010;26(1):50–7.
26. Chahla J, Cinque ME, Piuzzi NS, et al. A call for standardization in platelet-rich plasma preparation protocols and composition reporting: a systematic review of the clinical orthopaedic literature. J Bone Joint Surg Am 2017;99(20):1769–79.
27. Rodeo SA. Biologic approaches in sports medicine: potential, perils, and paths forward. Am J Sports Med 2016;44(7):1657–9.
28. Murray IR, Geeslin AG, Goudie EB, et al. Minimum information for studies evaluating biologics in orthopaedics (MIBO): platelet-rich plasma and mesenchymal stem cells. J Bone Joint Surg Am 2017;99(10):809–19.
29. Yeoh JC, Taylor BA. Osseous healing in foot and ankle surgery with autograft, allograft, and other orthobiologics. Orthop Clin North Am 2017;48(3):359–69.
30. Lin SS, Montemurro NJ, Krell ES. Orthobiologics in foot and ankle surgery. J Am Acad Orthop Surg 2016;24(2):113–22.
31. Kwong FN, Harris MB. Recent developments in the biology of fracture repair. J Am Acad Orthop Surg 2008;16(11):619–25.
32. Gross RH. The use of bone grafts and bone graft substitutes in pediatric orthopaedics: an overview. J Pediatr Orthop 2012;32:100–5.
33. Barnes GL, Kostenuik PJ, Gerstenfeld LC, et al. Growth factor regulation of fracture repair. J Bone Miner Res 1999;14(11):1805–15.
34. Lieberman JR, Daluiski A, Einhorn TA. The role of growth factors in the repair of bone. Biology and clinical applications. J Bone Joint Surg Am 2002;84-A(6):1032–44.
35. DiGiovanni CW, Lin SS, Baumhauer JF, et al, North American Orthopedic Foot and Ankle Study Group. Recombinant human platelet-derived growth factor-BB and beta-tricalcium phosphate (rhPDGF-BB/β-TCP): an alternative to autogenous bone graft. J Bone Joint Surg Am 2013;95(13):1184–92.
36. Bordei P. Locally applied platelet-derived growth factor accelerates fracture healing. J Bone Joint Surg Br 2011;93(12):1653–9.
37. Christersson A, Sandén B, Larsson S. Prospective randomized feasibility trial to assess the use of rhPDGF-BB in treatment of distal radius fractures. J Orthop Surg Res 2015;10:37.
38. Tokunaga T, Ide J, Arimura H, et al. Local application of gelatin hydrogel sheets impregnated with platelet-derived growth factor BB promotes tendon-to-bone healing after rotator cuff repair in rats. Arthroscopy 2015;31(8):1482–91.
39. Neer RM, Arnaud CD, Zanchetta JR, et al. Effect of parathyroid hormone (1-34) on fractures and bone mineral density in postmenopausal women with osteoporosis. N Engl J Med 2001;344(19):1434–41.
40. Hodsman AB, Bauer DC, Dempster DW, et al. Parathyroid hormone and teriparatide for the treatment of osteoporosis: a review of the evidence and suggested guidelines for its use. Endocr Rev 2005;26(5):688–703.
41. Alkhiary YM, Gerstenfeld LC, Krall E, et al. Enhancement of experimental fracture-healing by systemic administration of recombinant human parathyroid hormone (PTH 1-34). J Bone Joint Surg Am 2005;87(4):731–41.
42. Andreassen TT, Ejersted C, Oxlund H. Intermittent parathyroid hormone (1–34) treatment increases callus formation and mechanical strength of healing rat fractures. J Bone Miner Res 1999;14(6):960–8.
43. Komatsubara S, Mori S, Mashiba T, et al. Human parathyroid hormone (1-34) accelerates the fracture healing process of woven to lamellar bone replacement and new cortical shell formation in rat femora. Bone 2005;36(4):678–87.

44. Manabe T, Mori S, Mashiba T, et al. Human parathyroid hormone (1-34) accelerates natural fracture healing process in the femoral osteotomy model of cynomolgus monkeys. Bone 2007;40(6):1475–82.
45. Zhang W, Zhu J, Ma T, et al. Comparison of the effects of once-weekly and once-daily rhPTH (1-34) injections on promoting fracture healing in rodents. J Orthop Res 2017. https://doi.org/10.1002/jor.23750.
46. Aspenberg P, Genant HK, Johansson T, et al. Teriparatide for acceleration of fracture repair in humans: a prospective, randomized, double-blind study of 102 postmenopausal women with distal radial fractures. J Bone Miner Res 2010; 25(2):404–14.
47. Almirol EA, Chi LY, Khurana B, et al. Short-term effects of teriparatide versus placebo on bone biomarkers, structure, and fracture healing in women with lower-extremity stress fractures: a pilot study. J Clin Transl Endocrinol 2016;5:7–14.
48. Hettrich CM, Beamer BS, Bedi A, et al. The effect of rhPTH on the healing of tendon-to-bone in a rat model. J Orthop Res 2012;30(5):769–74.
49. Gorter EA, Hamdy NA, Appelman-Dijkstra NM, et al. The role of vitamin D in human fracture healing: a systematic review of the literature. Bone 2014;64:288–97.
50. Zhou S, Glowacki J, Kim SW, et al. Clinical characteristics influence in vitro action of 1,25-dihydroxyvitamin D(3) in human marrow stromal cells. J Bone Miner Res 2012;27(9):1992–2000.
51. van Leeuwen JP, van Driel M, van den Bemd GJ, et al. Vitamin D control of osteoblast function and bone extracellular matrix mineralization. Crit Rev Eukaryot Gene Expr 2001;11(1–3):199–226.
52. Flanagan AM, Stow MD, Kendall N, et al. The role of 1,25-dihydroxycholecalciferol and prostaglandin E2 in the regulation of human osteoclastic bone resorption in vitro. Int J Exp Pathol 1995;76(1):37–42.
53. Doetsch AM, Faber J, Lynnerup N, et al. The effect of calcium and vitamin D3 supplementation on the healing of the proximal humerus fracture: a randomized placebo-controlled study. Calcif Tissue Int 2004;75(3):183–8.
54. Kolb JP, Schilling AF, Bischoff J, et al. Calcium homeostasis influences radiological fracture healing in postmenopausal women. Arch Orthop Trauma Surg 2013; 133(2):187–92.
55. Avenell A, Mak JC, O'Connell D. Vitamin D and vitamin D analogues for preventing fractures in post-menopausal women and older men. Cochrane Database Syst Rev 2014;(4):CD000227.
56. Angeline ME, Ma R, Pascual-Garrido C, et al. Effect of diet-induced vitamin D deficiency on rotator cuff healing in a rat model. Am J Sports Med 2014;42(1): 27–34.
57. Gómez-Barrena E, Rosset P, Lozano D, et al. Bone fracture healing: cell therapy in delayed unions and nonunions. Bone 2015;70:93–101.
58. Taylor CJ. Delayed union and nonunion of fractures. In: Crenshaw AH, editor. Campbell's operative orthopaedics, vol. 28. St. Louis (MO): Mosby; 1992. p. 1287–345.
59. Jones AL, Bucholz RW, Bosse MJ, et al, BMP-2 Evaluation in Surgery for Tibial Trauma-Allgraft (BESTT-ALL) Study Group. Recombinant human BMP-2 and allograft compared with autogenous bone graft for reconstruction of diaphyseal tibial fractures with cortical defects. A randomized, controlled trial. J Bone Joint Surg Am 2006;88(7):1431–41.
60. Giannoudis PV, Kanakaris NK, Dimitriou R, et al. The synergistic effect of autograft and BMP-7 in the treatment of atrophic nonunions. Clin Orthop Relat Res 2009;467(12):3239–48.

61. Steiner ME, Murray MM, Rodeo SA. Strategies to improve anterior cruciate ligament healing and graft placement. Am J Sports Med 2008;36(1):176–89.
62. Rodeo SA, Arnoczky SP, Torzilli PA, et al. Tendon-healing in a bone tunnel. A biomechanical and histological study in the dog. J Bone Joint Surg Am 1993; 75(12):1795–803.
63. Ma CB, Kawamura S, Deng XH, et al. Bone morphogenetic proteins-signaling plays a role in tendon-to-bone healing: a study of rhBMP-2 and noggin. Am J Sports Med 2007;35(4):597–604.
64. Rodeo SA, Suzuki K, Deng XH, et al. Use of recombinant human bone morphogenetic protein-2 to enhance tendon healing in a bone tunnel. Am J Sports Med 1999;27(4):476–88.
65. Lui PP, Wong OT, Lee YW. Application of tendon-derived stem cell sheet for the promotion of graft healing in anterior cruciate ligament reconstruction. Am J Sports Med 2014;42(3):681–9.
66. Demirag B, Sarisozen B, Ozer O, et al. Enhancement of tendon-bone healing of anterior cruciate ligament grafts by blockage of matrix metalloproteinases. J Bone Joint Surg Am 2005;87(11):2401–10.
67. Rodeo SA, Potter HG, Kawamura S, et al. Biologic augmentation of rotator cuff tendon-healing with use of a mixture of osteoinductive growth factors. J Bone Joint Surg Am 2007;89(11):2485–97.
68. Kovacevic D, Gulotta LV, Ying L, et al. rhPDGF-BB promotes early healing in a rat rotator cuff repair model. Clin Orthop Relat Res 2015;473(5):1644–54.
69. Kovacevic D, Fox AJ, Bedi A, et al. Calcium-phosphate matrix with or without TGF-β3 improves tendon-bone healing after rotator cuff repair. Am J Sports Med 2011;39(4):811–9.
70. Zhao S, Peng L, Xie G, et al. Effect of the interposition of calcium phosphate materials on tendon-bone healing during repair of chronic rotator cuff tear. Am J Sports Med 2014;42(8):1920–9.
71. Rodeo SA, Kawamura S, Ma CB, et al. The effect of osteoclastic activity on tendon-to-bone healing: an experimental study in rabbits. J Bone Joint Surg Am 2007;89(10):2250–9.
72. Erickson BJ, Cvetanovich G, Waliullah K, et al. Two-stage revision anterior cruciate ligament reconstruction. Orthopedics 2016;39(3):e456–64.
73. Richter DL, Werner BC, Miller MD. Surgical pearls in revision anterior cruciate ligament surgery: when must I stage? Clin Sports Med 2017;36(1):173–87.
74. Werner BC, Gilmore CJ, Hamann JC, et al. Revision anterior cruciate ligament reconstruction: results of a single-stage approach using allograft dowel bone grafting for femoral defects. J Am Acad Orthop Surg 2016;24(8):581–7.
75. Tse BK, Vaughn ZD, Lindsey DP, et al. Evaluation of a one-stage ACL revision technique using bone void filler after cyclic loading. Knee 2012;19(4):477–81.
76. Chahla J, Dean CS, Cram TR, et al. Two-stage revision anterior cruciate ligament reconstruction: bone grafting technique using an allograft bone matrix. Arthrosc Tech 2016;5(1):e189–95.
77. Buyukdogan K, Laidlaw MS, Miller MD. Two-stage revision anterior cruciate ligament reconstruction using allograft bone dowels. Arthrosc Tech 2017;6(4): e1297–302.
78. Yamaguchi KT Jr, Mosich GM, Jones KJ. Arthroscopic delivery of injectable bone graft for staged revision anterior cruciate ligament reconstruction. Arthrosc Tech 2017;6(6):e2223–7.

79. Lash NJ, Feller JA, Batty LM, et al. Bone grafts and bone substitutes for opening-wedge osteotomies of the knee: a systematic review. Arthroscopy 2015;31(4): 720–30.
80. Giuseffi SA, Replogle WH, Shelton WR. Opening-wedge high tibial osteotomy: review of 100 consecutive cases. Arthroscopy 2015;31(11):2128–37.
81. Cameron JI, McCauley JC, Kermanshahi AY, et al. Lateral opening-wedge distal femoral osteotomy: pain relief, functional improvement, and survivorship at 5 years. Clin Orthop Relat Res 2015;473(6):2009–15.
82. Simon AM, Manigrasso MB, O'Connor JP. Cyclo-oxygenase 2 function is essential for bone fracture healing. J Bone Miner Res 2002;17(6):963–76.
83. Giannoudis PV, MacDonald DA, Matthews SJ, et al. Nonunion of the femoral diaphysis. The influence of reaming and non-steroidal anti-inflammatory drugs. J Bone Joint Surg Br 2000;82(5):655–8.
84. Sauerschnig M, Stolberg-Stolberg J, Schmidt C, et al. Effect of COX-2 inhibition on tendon-to-bone healing and PGE2 concentration after anterior cruciate ligament reconstruction. Eur J Med Res 2018;23(1):1.
85. Marquez-Lara A, Hutchinson ID, Nuñez F Jr, et al. Nonsteroidal anti-inflammatory drugs and bone-healing: a systematic review of research quality. JBJS Rev 2016; 4(3) [pii:01874474-201603000-00005].
86. Kim DH, Liu J, Bhat S, et al. Peroxisome proliferator-activated receptor delta agonist attenuates nicotine suppression effect on human mesenchymal stem cell-derived osteogenesis and involves increased expression of heme oxygenase-1. J Bone Miner Metab 2013;31(1):44–52.
87. Ng TK, Carballosa CM, Pelaez D, et al. Nicotine alters MicroRNA expression and hinders human adult stem cell regenerative potential. Stem Cells Dev 2013;22(5): 781–90.
88. Galatz LM, Silva MJ, Rothermich SY, et al. Nicotine delays tendon-to-bone healing in a rat shoulder model. J Bone Joint Surg Am 2006;88(9):2027–34.
89. Adams CI, Keating JF, Court-Brown CM. Cigarette smoking and open tibial fractures. Injury 2001;32(1):61–5.
90. Bender D, Jefferson-Keil T, Biglari B, et al. Cigarette smoking and its impact on fracture healing. Trauma 2013;16(1):18–22.
91. Moghaddam A, Weiss S, Wölfl CG, et al. Cigarette smoking decreases TGF-b1 serum concentrations after long bone fracture. Injury 2010;41(10):1020–5.
92. Scolaro JA, Schenker ML, Yannascoli S, et al. Cigarette smoking increases complications following fracture: a systematic review. J Bone Joint Surg Am 2014; 96(8):674–81.
93. Lee JJ, Patel R, Biermann JS, et al. The musculoskeletal effects of cigarette smoking. J Bone Joint Surg Am 2013;95(9):850–9.
94. Jiao H, Xiao E, Graves DT. Diabetes and its effect on bone and fracture healing. Curr Osteoporos Rep 2015;13(5):327–35.
95. Folk JW, Starr AJ, Early JS. Early wound complications of operative treatment of calcaneus fractures: analysis of 190 fractures. J Orthop Trauma 1999;13(5): 369–72.
96. Loder RT. The influence of diabetes mellitus on the healing of closed fractures. Clin Orthop Relat Res 1988;(232):210–6.
97. Bedi A, Fox AJ, Harris PE, et al. Diabetes mellitus impairs tendon-bone healing after rotator cuff repair. J Shoulder Elbow Surg 2010;19(7):978–88.

Ortho-Biologics for Ligament Repair and Reconstruction

Jorge Chahla, MD, PhD[a],*, Mitchell I. Kennedy, BS[b],
Zach S. Aman, BA[b], Robert F. LaPrade, MD, PhD[c]

KEYWORDS

- Platelet-rich plasma • Anterior cruciate ligament • Growth factor
- Transforming growth factor • Bone marrow aspirate concentrate

KEY POINTS

- Despite the recent appraisal of biologics within treatment protocols, no clear algorithm for indication, processing methodology, or application exists currently.
- There is a significant potential for enhancement of tissue healing within both acute and chronic conditions in restoring native or near native tissue.
- Biologics may provide an alternative to surgical intervention when nonoperative treatment is preferred by patients or surgeons.
- When biologics are used in addition to surgical intervention, there is a potential for enhanced bone mineral density, bone volume, overall graft integrity, and vascularity within cells.
- Currently, the literature is inconsistent in providing definite conclusions on outcomes and usage of biologics for the treatment of musculoskeletal injuries; but laboratory, animal, and some clinical studies have provided promising results for the future direction of orthopedic treatment protocols and rehabilitation.

INTRODUCTION

Novelties and technology improvement for ortho-biological therapies, tissue grafting, and surgical augmentation have exhibited overwhelming growth in the past decade.[1] At first, biologics were envisioned to enhance tissue healing in both acute and chronic conditions by stimulating the recovery processes to restore native or near-native tissue while reducing risks for treatment failure. Nonetheless, symptom

Disclosure Statement: The authors have nothing to disclose.
[a] Sports Medicne and Shoulder Service, Midwest Orthopaedics at Rush, 1611 Harrison Avenue, Suite 300, Chicago, IL 60612, USA; [b] The Steadman Philippon Research Institute, 181 West Meadow Drive, Suite 400, Vail, CO 81657, USA; [c] The Steadman Clinic, 181 West Meadow Drive, Suite 400, Vail, CO 81657, USA
* Corresponding author. 181 West Meadow Drive, Suite 400, Vail, CO 81657.
E-mail address: jachahla@msn.com

Clin Sports Med 38 (2019) 97–107
https://doi.org/10.1016/j.csm.2018.08.003
0278-5919/19/© 2018 Elsevier Inc. All rights reserved.

sportsmed.theclinics.com

management has recently become another important indication for their use.[2–4] The most popular biological modalities currently used for the treatment of acute and chronic musculoskeletal conditions and as adjuvants for conservative and surgical approaches include hyaluronic acid, single/combined growth factors (GFs) therapy, platelet-rich plasma (PRP) (**Figs. 1** and **2**), and bone marrow aspirate concentrate (BMAC) (**Fig. 3**).

However, despite the upsurge on the use and reported success of many of these therapies, there is no clear algorithm for the indications, processing methodology, application, and reporting that has led to inconsistencies in clinical and basic science results.[5–7] Hence, establishing an optimal protocol for the treatment of various musculoskeletal entities remains a challenge because the specific treatment or combination of them, the number of applications, the processing method, and the real and long-term efficacy of these biological approaches has yet to be determined.[8,9]

Complex biomechanics, different vectors of load, and an intra-articular hostile environment have also been reported as serious obstacles to successfully adhere tissue-engineered and autologous biologics to damaged tissue, regenerate homogeneous tissue, and finally revascularize the tissue sufficiently and timely to prevent a future reinjury.[10–12] For the aforementioned reasons, the purpose of this article is to review current concepts on several biological treatment approaches as an adjuvant for the most commonly performed ligament injuries repair or reconstructions.

KNEE
Anterior Cruciate Ligament

Despite being one of the most frequent procedures in orthopedics (reported to be the sixth most common),[13] limited progress has been made to improve anterior cruciate ligament (ACL) reconstruction and its healing capacity or to improve the time of ACL graft ligament incorporation to enhance knee biomechanics, reduce the return to sports times, and ultimately limit the development of degenerative joint changes.[14–17]

In this regard, regenerative treatment protocols are thought to have the potential to improve current surgical ACL interventions by enhancing graft incorporation and

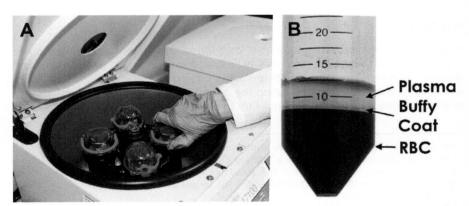

Fig. 1. (*A*) The centrifuge setup for processing of PRP and (*B*) the final result with 3 distinct layers of cellular material after processing the sample. At the top of the test tube is the platelet-poor plasma; beneath this layer is the buffy coat where most platelets lie (the deepest layer of the buffy coat layer contains high concentrations of white blood cells), and at the bottom layer are the red blood cells (RBCs).

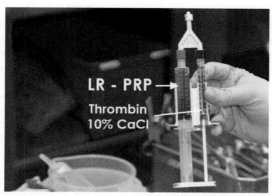

Fig. 2. A double syringe system for injection (11:1 ratio allowing homologous mixture of the PRP [*left*] and a gelling agent solution [*right*], respectively). Gelling agent solution typically consists of thrombin and 10% calcium chloride (CaCl) solution (1000 IUs thrombin:1 mL CaCl). LR, leukocyte rich.

strength, gene activation, trophic induction, and microenvironment facilitation and signaling with cells or bioactive factors to optimize, delay, or prevent premature progression of osteoarthritis.[18] It is accepted that the success of an ACL reconstruction depends heavily on biological processes for each phase of the healing process. Commonly reported regenerative modalities contain various GFs, including transforming GF β-1 (TGF-β1), fibroblast GF-2 (FGF-2), insulinlike GF, epidermal GF, platelet-derived GF (PDGF), and vascular endothelial GF (VEGF). These GFs have demonstrated positive effects on cell proliferation, cell migration, angiogenesis, and extracellular matrix (ECM) production in numerous cell types of both in vivo and in vitro models.[19]

The primary cell in the ACL is the fibroblast. The fibroblast has receptors for many of these GFs, including PDGF, TGF-β, and FGF. For example, PDGF stimulates fibroblast growth, migration, and biosynthetic activity,[20] which could promote an improved ligamentization of the graft used for ACL repair or reconstruction and minimize the proinflammatory factors released immediately after surgery but might also contribute to a better and faster integration of the graft within the femoral and tibial tunnels, thus, avoiding an increased failure risk.[21]

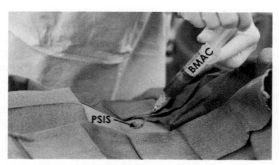

Fig. 3. A patient in ventral decubitus for BMAC from the left posterior superior iliac spine (PSIS).

Preclinical studies

Important basic science studies have been performed in the area of ligament healing in an attempt to regenerate/repair ligaments in a less invasive approach using the tissue remnants available. Although in clinical practice this is not often possible, because of the lack of viable tissue pending the severity and/or chronicity of the injury, growing preclinical work has provided the basis to improve these biological approaches. GFs, such as TGF-β1,[22] FGF-2,[23] and basic-FGF,[24] have been reported to regulate and improve cellular activities and proliferation and ECM deposition and to influence the differentiation of mesenchymal stem cells (MSCs) into fibroblasts in the repair process of torn ligaments. Particularly, the GFs outlined later have exhibited positive effects on various biological processes needed to improve ACL healing.

The TGF-β family is a key regulator during embryologic development and also plays a significant role in the early modulation of scar tissue formation during connective tissue healing.[25] Studies comparing the application of different GFs in animals with partial ACL tears and ACL explant models suggested that TGF-β1 might stimulate initial healing and overall healing both histologically and biomechanically.[26,27] Kondo and colleagues[26] reported on the effect of TGF- β1 in a rabbit ACL injury model and reported significant improvement of the biomechanical and histologic healing properties of injured ACLs treated with TGF-β1 when compared with controls. Recently, it has been reported that blocking VEGF reduces angiogenesis, graft maturation, and biomechanical strength following an ACL reconstruction in a rat model.[28] Further, a different group studied 18 sheep undergoing ACL reconstruction with either a VEGF-augmented graft or a control group. The VEGF group demonstrated improved vascularization and fibroblast infiltration; however, increased graft laxity was found at 12 weeks.[29]

Murray and colleagues[30] reported on a porcine ACL repair model using clotted PRP, suggesting that there was no beneficial effect of adding PRP when compared with controls. It was theorized that the fibrin clot containing the platelets may have been prematurely dissolved in the intra-articular environment by circulating plasmin in the synovial fluid.

These findings directed the attention to developing scaffolds to protect the graft from early degradation due to the hostile intra-articular environment. Consequently, Cheng and colleagues[31] showed that the addition of PRP to a collagen hydrogel resulted in a significantly increased cellular metabolic activity, reduced apoptotic rate, and stimulation of collagen production in the cells from the immature and adolescent animals but had less effect on adult cells animals.

A study using a rat model compared ACL regeneration between animal groups subjected to intra-articular injection of fresh whole bone marrow cells (BMCs), cultured MSCs, or saline in partial ACL tears.[32] The investigators suggested that intra-articular bone marrow transplantation using fresh whole BMCs is an effective treatment of ACL partial rupture and reported nearly normal strength and ligament healing compared with control subjects. Similarly, Kanaya and colleagues[33] reported that intra-articular injection of MSCs resulted in a healed ligament with superior histologic scores and a greater failure load compared with nontreated control knees. A recent study by Lui and colleagues[34] compared ACL reconstructions with tendon-derived stem cell sheets (after treatment with connective tissue GF) and a control group in 97 rats. The treatment arm exhibited higher tunnel bone mineral density and bone volume, better graft osteointegration, and higher intra-articular graft integrity with lower cellularity, vascularity, and cell alignment compared with the control group.

Clinical studies

Improvements in tissue engineering and regenerative medicine technology have resulted in a new interest in the biological augmentation of ACL repairs and reconstructions, including GF, PRP, stem cells, and bio-scaffolds. A recent systematic review[35] reported on 23 studies, including one reporting on stem cells, one on concomitant application of PRP and stem cells, and 21 articles on PRP. Two studies reported on ACL repair with biologics and the remaining 21 on ACL reconstruction augmented with PRP. The investigators concluded that the role of PRP on ACL repair/reconstruction is still controversial and is only related to improved graft maturation over time, without beneficial effects in terms of clinical outcome, bone-graft integration, and prevention of bony tunnel enlargement in the short-term outcome.

Seijas and colleagues[36] reported on 19 professional soccer players with partial ACL tears treated with intraligamentous placement of PDGFs into the intact bundle. Eighteen of 19 players were able to return to their previous level of play at a mean of 16.20 weeks. Platelet-rich GF (PRGF-Endoret)[37] was applied in the intact posterolateral bundle intra-articularly in a different study by Anitua and colleagues.[37] No complications and satisfactory objective results (KT-1000; MEDMETRIC, San Diego, CA) were reported in this study, and postoperative MRI evaluation demonstrated complete ligamentization at 1 year after surgery with good anatomic arrangement.

Radice and colleagues[38] reported on 100 ACL reconstructions prospectively, comparing PRP gel (PRPG) with a control group. Notably, graft homogeneity was 48% shorter in the PRPG group (179 vs 369 days). Additionally, Vogrin and colleagues[39] reported on 50 patients (25 thrombin-activated PRP-soaked grafts and 25 control group) and demonstrated improved anterior-posterior instrumented knee stability via a KT-2000 (MEDMETRIC; San Diego, CA) arthrometer at 6 months. Conversely, Nin and colleagues[40] reported on 100 patients undergoing an ACL reconstruction with bone-tendon-bone allograft (double-blind randomized clinical trial). The investigators reported no difference was found in terms of subjective outcome, biomechanical integration, or graft integration at 2 years' follow-up.

Gobbi and colleagues[41] evaluated the 5-year clinical results of PRP injection in 58 athletes treated by ACL suture repair in addition to microfracture of the intercondylar notch. They reported that 78% of the patients returned to their sports activities. The side-to-side difference in anterior translation significantly decreased from 4.1 mm (SD = 1.6) preoperatively to 1.4 mm (SD = 0.8) postoperatively ($P < .05$). Four patients had a retear during sporting activity and underwent an ACL reconstruction within 2 years from the primary repair surgery. This case series concluded that PRP injection was effective in restoring knee stability and function in young individuals with acute partial ACL tears.

Limited evidence exists on histologic data for PRP application after ACL reconstruction. Sanchez and colleagues[42] compared PRGF-assisted ACL reconstructions versus nonaugmented ACL reconstructions that required a second-look arthroscopy (loose body or hardware removal, meniscal tears treatment, or cyclops lesions resection) at a minimum of 6 months. Although gross morphology demonstrated no difference, histologically, newly formed connective tissue enveloping the graft was found in 77.3% of the intervention group versus 40.0% of control subjects.

Concerning BMAC application as an adjuvant for ACL surgery, Centeno and colleagues[43] reported on 10 patients with ACL tears treated with an intraligamentous injection of autologous bone marrow concentrate and PRP using fluoroscopic guidance. ACL laxity and MRI evidence of a grade I, II (partial), or III (complete) tears were documented (always with <1 cm retraction of the ACL stump). ACL tears were assessed by MRI, and software was used to objectively quantify changes of ligament integrity through 5 different types of measurements of ACL pixel intensity. Seven of 10 patients showed improvement in at least 4 of these 5 objective MRI measures. The mean visual analog scale change decreased by 1.7 ($P = .25$), and the mean Lower Extremity Functional Scale increased by 23.3 ($P = .03$); a mean improvement of 86.7% was reported.

Medial Collateral Ligament

Isolated medial collateral ligament (MCL) injuries are the most common knee ligament injuries and are typically managed with conservative treatment resulting in satisfactory results. However, mechanical and histologic properties typically do not return to normal.[44,45] For this reason, the use of PRP to advance MCL healing has been proposed.[46]

Preclinical studies
Despite the frequent use of PRP to treat ligamentous injuries, there is limited information on the use of PRP in basic science; clinical trials to determine if improvement can be achieved for biomechanics or ligamentous healing can be accelerated.[47] LaPrade and colleagues[48] reported that one single dose of either PPP or a 2-times dose of PRP at the time of injury did not accelerate ligament healing (**Fig. 4**). Additionally, a 4-times dose of PRP demonstrated a significant negative effect on ligament strength and collagen orientation (relative to the sham group) at 6 weeks after injury. The investigators concluded that MCL tears treated with PRP immediately after injury or surgery may not improve healing at low doses of PRP and could be harming ligament healing at higher PRP doses. In a biomechanical analysis, Yoshioka and colleagues[49] reported significantly improved structural properties of MCLs in rabbits treated with leukocyte-reduced PRP relative to controls. However, no analysis was performed taking the native ligament biomechanical properties; only a comparison between the PRGF and untreated group was made.

Clinical studies
Literature on the beneficial effect of PRP treatment of MCL injuries is limited. Only one level IV case study report has evaluated the clinical use of PRP with outcomes of isolated grade II MCL injuries.[50] Eirale and colleagues[50] described a successful case of a competitive soccer player in which they opted for conservative treatment with multiple PRP injections and rehabilitation. The athlete returned to play after 18 days with excellent functional scores and without symptoms, but radiological imaging showed

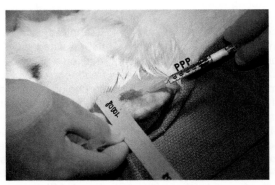

Fig. 4. A rabbit MCL being injected with PPP after creating a grade III tear to the ligament to determine the effect of different concentrations of platelets in MCL healing.

incomplete healing of the ligament.[50] Despite this, the athlete had no recurrence of injury or further complications at 16 months' follow-up.[50] This study gives evidence that PRP may play a role in MCL healing with conservative treatment; however, it is encouraged that further clinical outcome studies be performed to elucidate the value of PRP with MCL injury.

Ulnar Collateral Ligament of the Elbow

Enhancing the treatment options for ulnar collateral ligament (UCL) deficiency has long been of interest in the world of sports medicine. Highly prevalent among overhead-throwing athletes, primarily with baseball pitchers from youth to professional levels, improved UCL reconstruction techniques have resulted in increased return-to-play rates between 53% and 90% after once being thought of as a career-ending injury.[51–56] However, there is a disparity in the literature on the postoperative UCL reconstruction outcomes because it has been reported that 3% to 40% of surgical re-constructions result in complications.[57–60] Although there is a multitude of factors that influence UCL recovery, adjunctive treatments like PRP and MSCs may accelerate the timetable for athletes returning to sport and improve overall outcomes. Additionally, biological injections could possibly serve as a nonoperative treatment, acting to bypass a year-long recovery period and pose as an alternative to the perceptually adhered to Tommy John surgery.[56,61,62]

Preclinical studies

To the authors' knowledge, no preclinical studies have been performed specifically evaluating the use of biologics for UCL healing. Because of the potential therapeutic use that has been seen for ACL, rotator cuff, and Achilles tendon injury in animal models, it is thought that PRP and MSCs can be applied to UCL injury and are frequently used in clinical settings.

Clinical studies

Two studies have used biological adjuncts for nonoperative treatment of a partial UCL tear with promising results, in contrast to clinical outcomes seen in other joints.[59,63] In a case series of overhead-throwing athletes, Podesta and colleagues[63] reported that 88% of athletes with partial UCL tears returned to normal levels of play at 12 weeks after a single PRP injection. Along with satisfying functionality, the investigators also reported decreased medial elbow joint space on valgus loading.[63] Furthermore, another study of 44 competitive baseball players reported that 73% of athletes had good to excellent results following a PRP injection when supplemented with a return-to-play rehabilitation program.[59] Unfortunately, no clinical studies of conserva-tive management of complete UCL injuries with MSCs or scaffolds have been pub-lished.[62] However, with the increasing popularity of these methods for treatment of shoulder and knee joint injuries, it should be expected that MSCs and scaffolds would serve a significant role in future UCL treatment techniques.

SUMMARY OF RECOMMENDATIONS

In recent literature, biologics have been shown to have positive results in improving tissue regeneration in laboratory and animal studies; but in the clinical setting, results are mixed in demonstrating its efficacy for patient care. The use of PRP has been tested in both forms of rehabilitation following surgery as well as a replacement to liga-mentous reconstructions for patients/surgeons wishing to avoid surgical intervention, but outcomes are clouded among beneficial and neutral effects. With more consistent results of MSC and PRP effects on patient outcomes (preferably with objective data, such as imaging or histology), the future direction of orthopedic treatment may continue to progress further into less invasive procedures.

REFERENCES

1. Doral MN, Tandoğan RN, Mann G, et al. Sports injuries: prevention, diagnosis, treatment and rehabilitation. Verlag Berlin, Heidelberg: Springer; 2011.
2. Toolan BC. Current concepts review: orthobiologics. Foot Ankle Int 2006;27(7): 561–6.
3. Goodman SB, Yao Z, Keeney M, et al. The future of biologic coatings for orthopaedic implants. Biomaterials 2013;34(13):3174–83.
4. LaPrade RF, Geeslin AG, Murray IR, et al. Biologic treatments for sports injuries II think tank–current concepts, future research, and barriers to advancement, part 1: biologics overview, ligament injury, tendinopathy. Am J Sports Med 2016; 44(12):3270–83.
5. DeLong JM, Russell RP, Mazzocca AD. Platelet-rich plasma: the PAW classification system. Arthroscopy 2012;28(7):998–1009.
6. Dohan Ehrenfest DMA I, Zumstein MA, Zhang CQ, et al. Classification of platelet concentrates (Platelet-Rich Plasma-PRP, Platelet-Rich Fibrin-PRF) for topical and infiltrative use in orthopedic and sports medicine: current consensus, clinical implications and perspectives. Muscles Ligaments Tendons J 2014;4(1):3–9.
7. Holton J, Imam M, Ward J, et al. The basic science of bone marrow aspirate concentrate in chondral injuries. Orthop Rev (Pavia) 2016;8(3):6659.
8. Foster TE, Puskas BL, Mandelbaum BR, et al. Platelet-rich plasma: from basic science to clinical applications. Am J Sports Med 2009;37(11):2259–72.
9. Sheth U, Simunovic N, Klein G, et al. Efficacy of autologous platelet-rich plasma use for orthopaedic indications: a meta-analysis. J Bone Joint Surg Am 2012; 94(4):298–307.
10. Zhang L, Hu J, Athanasiou KA. The role of tissue engineering in articular cartilage repair and regeneration. Crit Rev Biomed Eng 2009;37(1–2):1–57.
11. Amini AR, Laurencin CT, Nukavarapu SP. Bone tissue engineering: recent advances and challenges. Crit Rev Biomed Eng 2012;40(5):363–408.
12. Frohlich M, Grayson WL, Wan LQ, et al. Tissue engineered bone grafts: biological requirements, tissue culture and clinical relevance. Curr Stem Cell Res Ther 2008;3(4):254–64.
13. Garrett WE Jr, Swiontkowski MF, Weinstein JN, et al. American Board of Orthopaedic Surgery Practice of the Orthopaedic Surgeon: part-II, certification examination case mix. J Bone Joint Surg Am 2006;88(3):660–7.
14. Brown CH Jr, Carson EW. Revision anterior cruciate ligament surgery. Clin Sports Med 1999;18(1):109–71.
15. Gottlob CA, Baker CL Jr, Pellissier JM, et al. Cost effectiveness of anterior cruciate ligament reconstruction in young adults. Clin Orthop Relat Res 1999;(367): 272–82.
16. Kim S, Bosque J, Meehan JP, et al. Increase in outpatient knee arthroscopy in the United States: a comparison of National Surveys of Ambulatory Surgery, 1996 and 2006. J Bone Joint Surg Am 2011;93(11):994–1000.
17. Spindler KP, Wright RW. Clinical practice. Anterior cruciate ligament tear. N Engl J Med 2008;359(20):2135–42.
18. Kiapour AM, Murray MM. Basic science of anterior cruciate ligament injury and repair. Bone Joint Res 2014;3(2):20–31.

19. Hutchinson ID, Rodeo SA, Perrone GS, et al. Can platelet-rich plasma enhance anterior cruciate ligament and meniscal repair? J Knee Surg 2015;28(1):19–28.
20. Molloy T, Wang Y, Murrell G. The roles of growth factors in tendon and ligament healing. Sports Med 2003;33(5):381–94.
21. Andriolo L, Di Matteo B, Kon E, et al. PRP augmentation for ACL reconstruction. Biomed Res Int 2015;2015:371746.
22. Xie J, Wang C, Huang DY, et al. TGF-beta1 induces the different expressions of lysyl oxidases and matrix metalloproteinases in anterior cruciate ligament and medial collateral ligament fibroblasts after mechanical injury. J Biomech 2013; 46(5):890–8.
23. Madry H, Kohn D, Cucchiarini M. Direct FGF-2 gene transfer via recombinant adeno-associated virus vectors stimulates cell proliferation, collagen production, and the repair of experimental lesions in the human ACL. Am J Sports Med 2013; 41(1):194–202.
24. Kobayashi D, Kurosaka M, Yoshiya S, et al. Effect of basic fibroblast growth factor on the healing of defects in the canine anterior cruciate ligament. Knee Surg Sports Traumatol Arthrosc 1997;5(3):189–94.
25. Muller B, Bowman KF Jr, Bedi A. ACL graft healing and biologics. Clin Sports Med 2013;32(1):93–109.
26. Kondo E, Yasuda K, Yamanaka M, et al. Effects of administration of exogenous growth factors on biomechanical properties of the elongation-type anterior cruciate ligament injury with partial laceration. Am J Sports Med 2005;33(2):188–96.
27. Spindler KP, Imro AK, Mayes CE, et al. Patellar tendon and anterior cruciate ligament have different mitogenic responses to platelet-derived growth factor and transforming growth factor beta. J Orthop Res 1996;14(4):542–6.
28. Takayama K, Kawakami Y, Mifune Y, et al. The effect of blocking angiogenesis on anterior cruciate ligament healing following stem cell transplantation. Biomaterials 2015;60:9–19.
29. Yoshikawa T, Tohyama H, Katsura T, et al. Effects of local administration of vascular endothelial growth factor on mechanical characteristics of the semitendinosus tendon graft after anterior cruciate ligament reconstruction in sheep. Am J Sports Med 2006;34(12):1918–25.
30. Murray MM, Palmer M, Abreu E, et al. Platelet-rich plasma alone is not sufficient to enhance suture repair of the ACL in skeletally immature animals: an in vivo study. J Orthop Res 2009;27(5):639–45.
31. Cheng M, Johnson VM, Murray MM. Effects of age and platelet-rich plasma on ACL cell viability and collagen gene expression. J Orthop Res 2012;30(1):79–85.
32. Oe K, Kushida T, Okamoto N, et al. New strategies for anterior cruciate ligament partial rupture using bone marrow transplantation in rats. Stem Cell Dev 2011; 20(4):671–9.
33. Kanaya A, Deie M, Adachi N, et al. Intra-articular injection of mesenchymal stromal cells in partially torn anterior cruciate ligaments in a rat model. Arthroscopy 2007;23(6):610–7.
34. Lui PP, Wong OT, Lee YW. Application of tendon-derived stem cell sheet for the promotion of graft healing in anterior cruciate ligament reconstruction. Am J Sports Med 2014;42(3):681–9.
35. Di Matteo B, Kon E, Filardo G. Intra-articular platelet-rich plasma for the treatment of osteoarthritis. Ann Transl Med 2016;4(3):63.
36. Seijas R, Ares O, Cusco X, et al. Partial anterior cruciate ligament tears treated with intraligamentary plasma rich in growth factors. World J Orthop 2014;5(3): 373–8.

37. Anitua E. Plasma rich in growth factors: preliminary results of use in the preparation of future sites for implants. Int J Oral Maxillofac Implants 1999;14(4):529–35.

38. Radice F, Yanez R, Gutierrez V, et al. Comparison of magnetic resonance imaging findings in anterior cruciate ligament grafts with and without autologous platelet-derived growth factors. Arthroscopy 2010;26(1):50–7.

39. Vogrin M, Rupreht M, Crnjac A, et al. The effect of platelet-derived growth factors on knee stability after anterior cruciate ligament reconstruction: a prospective randomized clinical study. Wien Klin Wochenschr 2010;122(Suppl 2):91–5.

40. Nin JR, Gasque GM, Azcarate AV, et al. Has platelet-rich plasma any role in anterior cruciate ligament allograft healing? Arthroscopy 2009;25(11):1206–13.

41. Gobbi A, Karnatzikos G, Sankineani SR, et al. Biological augmentation of ACL refixation in partial lesions in a group of athletes: results at the 5-year follow-up. Tech Orthop 2013;28(2):180–4.

42. Sanchez M, Anitua E, Azofra J, et al. Ligamentization of tendon grafts treated with an endogenous preparation rich in growth factors: gross morphology and histology. Arthroscopy 2010;26(4):470–80.

43. Centeno CJ, Pitts J, Al-Sayegh H, et al. Anterior cruciate ligament tears treated with percutaneous injection of autologous bone marrow nucleated cells: a case series. J Pain Res 2015;8:437–47.

44. Niyibizi C, Kavalkovich K, Yamaji T, et al. Type V collagen is increased during rabbit medial collateral ligament healing. Knee Surg Sports Traumatol Arthrosc 2000; 8(5):281–5.

45. Scheffler SU, Clineff TD, Papageorgiou CD, et al. Structure and function of the healing medial collateral ligament in a goat model. Ann Biomed Eng 2001; 29(2):173–80.

46. Andia I, Maffulli N. Use of platelet-rich plasma for patellar tendon and medial collateral ligament injuries: best current clinical practice. J Knee Surg 2015; 28(1):11–8.

47. Engebretsen L, Steffen K, Alsousou J, et al. IOC consensus paper on the use of platelet-rich plasma in sports medicine. Br J Sports Med 2010;44(15):1072–81.

48. LaPrade RF, Goodrich LR, Philipps J, et al. Use of platelet-rich plasma immediately post-injury to improve ligament healing was not successful in an in vivo animal model. Am J Sports Med 2018;46(3):702–12.

49. Yoshioka T, Kanamori A, Washio T, et al. The effects of plasma rich in growth factors (PRGF-Endoret) on healing of medial collateral ligament of the knee. Knee Surg Sports Traumatol Arthrosc 2013;21(8):1763–9.

50. Eirale C, Mauri E, Hamilton B. Use of platelet rich plasma in an isolated complete medial collateral ligament lesion in a professional football (soccer) player: a case report. Asian J Sports Med 2013;4(2):158–62.

51. Erickson BJ, Gupta AK, Harris JD, et al. Rate of return to pitching and performance after Tommy John surgery in Major League Baseball pitchers. Am J Sports Med 2014;42(3):536–43.

52. Makhni EC, Lee RW, Morrow ZS, et al. Performance, return to competition, and reinjury after tommy john surgery in major league baseball pitchers: a review of 147 cases. Am J Sports Med 2014;42(6):1323–32.

53. Osbahr DC, Cain EL Jr, Raines BT, et al. Long-term outcomes after ulnar collateral ligament reconstruction in competitive baseball players: minimum 10-year follow-up. Am J Sports Med 2014;42(6):1333–42.

54. Park JY, Oh KS, Bahng SC, et al. Does well maintained graft provide consistent return to play after medial ulnar collateral ligament reconstruction of the elbow joint in elite baseball players? Clin Orthop Surg 2014;6(2):190–5.

55. Rohrbough JT, Altchek DW, Hyman J, et al. Medial collateral ligament reconstruction of the elbow using the docking technique. Am J Sports Med 2002;30(4): 541–8.
56. Jobe FW, Stark H, Lombardo SJ. Reconstruction of the ulnar collateral ligament in athletes. J Bone Joint Surg Am 1986;68(8):1158–63.
57. Conway JE, Jobe FW, Glousman RE, et al. Medial instability of the elbow in throwing athletes. Treatment by repair or reconstruction of the ulnar collateral ligament. J Bone Joint Surg Am 1992;74(1):67–83.
58. Dodson CC, Thomas A, Dines JS, et al. Medial ulnar collateral ligament reconstruction of the elbow in throwing athletes. Am J Sports Med 2006;34(12): 1926–32.
59. Dines JS, Williams PN, ElAttrache N, et al. Platelet-rich plasma can be used to successfully treat elbow ulnar collateral ligament insufficiency in high-level throwers. Am J Orthop (Belle Mead NJ) 2016;45(5):296–300.
60. Azar FM, Andrews JR, Wilk KE, et al. Operative treatment of ulnar collateral ligament injuries of the elbow in athletes. Am J Sports Med 2000;28(1):16–23.
61. Ahmad CS, Grantham WJ, Greiwe RM. Public perceptions of Tommy John surgery. Phys Sportsmed 2012;40(2):64–72.
62. Rebolledo BJ, Dugas JR, Bedi A, et al. Avoiding Tommy John Surgery: what are the alternatives? Am J Sports Med 2017;45(13):3143–8.
63. Podesta L, Crow SA, Volkmer D, et al. Treatment of partial ulnar collateral ligament tears in the elbow with platelet-rich plasma. Am J Sports Med 2013;41(7): 1689–94.

Orthobiologics for Focal Articular Cartilage Defects

Taylor M. Southworth, BS[a], Neal B. Naveen, BS[a],
Benedict U. Nwachukwu, MD, MBA[a], Brian J. Cole, MD, MBA[a],
Rachel M. Frank, MD[b],*

KEYWORDS

- Cartilage restoration • Stem cells • Orthobiologics • PRP • Cartilage defect
- Cartilage transplant

KEY POINTS

- Focal chondral defects of the knee are very common, and often result in pain, dysfunction, and in many cases, joint deterioration, and ultimately, the development of osteoarthritis.
- Because of the limitations of conventional treatments, biologic augmentation for the treatment of focal cartilage defects has recently become an area of interest.
- Orthobiologics for focal chondral defects can be applied in the clinical setting, as an isolated surgical procedure, or as an augment to cartilage restoration surgery.
- Orthobiologics used for cartilage defects include (but are not limited to) bone marrow aspirate concentrate, adipose-derived mesenchymal stem cells, platelet-rich plasma, and micronized allogeneic cartilage.

INTRODUCTION

Orthobiologics have become increasingly recognized as treatment options for a variety of orthopedic pathologies. Orthobiologics are currently being used as treatments for osteoarthritis (OA),[1–4] lateral epicondylitis,[5,6] fracture healing,[7] ligament reconstruction,[8] and focal articular cartilage defects.[9–13] Examples of orthobiologics include platelet-rich plasma (PRP), bone marrow aspirate concentrate (BMAC), amniotic membrane–derived mesenchymal stem cells (MSC), and adipose-derived MSCs.

Disclosure Statement: R.M. Frank has nothing to disclose. Dr B.J. Cole receives financial or research support from the following: Arthrex, DJ Orthopedics, Elsevier Publishing, Arthrex, Inc, Flexion, Regentis, Smith and Nephew, Zimmer, Aqua Boom, Biomerix, Giteliscope, Ossio, Aesculap/B.Braun, Geistlich, National Institutes of Health (NIAMS & NICHD), Sanofi-Aventis, Athletico, JRF Ortho, Tornier.
[a] Department of Orthopedics, Rush University Medical Center, 1611 West Harrison, Suite 300, Chicago, IL 60612, USA; [b] Sports Medicine and Shoulder Surgery, Department of Orthopaedic Surgery, University of Colorado School of Medicine, 12631 East 17th Avenue, Mail Stop B202, Aurora, CO 80045, USA
* Corresponding author.
E-mail address: rachel.frank@ucdenver.edu

Clin Sports Med 38 (2019) 109–122
https://doi.org/10.1016/j.csm.2018.09.001
0278-5919/19/© 2018 Elsevier Inc. All rights reserved.

sportsmed.theclinics.com

There is a limited amount of literature assessing the efficacy of these techniques as treatment of focal articular cartilage defects. This article aims to discuss the current research and recommendations available on the use of orthobiologics for the treatment of focal articular cartilage defects.

BACKGROUND

Focal articular cartilage defects are common in the knee, and many times result in pain, swelling, and overall joint dysfunction. Widuchowski and colleagues[14] found the prevalence of chondral lesions in the knee to be 60% of those undergoing arthroscopies. Of these, 67% were classified as localized focal osteochondral lesions. Another study showed 63% of patients undergoing knee arthroscopies exhibited chondral lesions.[15] Although focal articular cartilage defects appear to be less prevalent in other joints such as the glenohumeral joint at 5% to 17%,[16] they can still be a substantial source of pain and discomfort. In addition, studies have suggested that focal cartilage lesions may progress to OA,[17] a major cause of morbidity in the United States.[18] Guettler and colleagues[19] examined the altered loading patterns and rim stress concentrations corresponding to different defect sizes and found that in lesions larger than 10 mm, the decreased contact area, increased rim stress, and increased stress on the surrounding cartilage are likely a few of the factors leading to degeneration of the remaining cartilage and, ultimately, arthritis.

Because of its aneural and avascular environment, articular cartilage lacks the ability to heal spontaneously. For this reason, combined with the symptomatic nature of the lesions and the predisposition for OA, early intervention is recommended to restore joint function and pressure distribution. The ultimate goal for treatment of chondral and osteochondral defects is to regenerate natural hyaline cartilage that is well integrated with the surrounding uninjured cartilage. Treatment of these lesions with orthobiologics can be performed either as an isolated injection-based treatment in the clinical or surgical setting, as described throughout the other articles in this text, or during surgery via augmentation of another cartilage restoration technique. Cartilage restoration surgery can be classified into 3 main categories. The first is palliative surgery, which consists of arthroscopic debridement, chondroplasty, and/or lavage. The second is reparative surgery, which includes marrow stimulation techniques, such as a microfracture, with or without biologic augmentation, and the third is restorative, which encompasses osteochondral grafting, including autograft or allograft, as well as autologous chondrocyte implantation (ACI) as well as matrix-induced ACI (MACI).[20]

Marrow stimulation techniques have traditionally been recommended for focal full-thickness chondral lesions less than 2 cm, or in patients with lesions greater than 3 cm and a modest level of physical demand.[20] This procedure functions to stimulate the subchondral bone marrow by creating a blood clot within the lesion rich with marrow elements, including MSCs for healing and fibrocartilage formation. Microfracture has shown its optimal results in patients who are less than 45 years old with lesions less than 2 cm, and a body mass index of less than 30,[21] suggesting it is not an effective treatment in older patients and those with larger lesions. In addition, microfracture leads to the growth of fibrocartilage, which is less durable than hyaline cartilage. Because of these limitations, biologic augmentation of microfracture for treatment of focal cartilage defects has recently become an area of interest.

ACI uses a 2-step surgical procedure in order to implant the patient's own chondrocytes into the defect.[22] The first step is an arthroscopic biopsy of a nonarticulating area of the knee to obtain healthy chondrocytes for culture. The second surgery involves the implantation of these cultured chondrocytes after about 3 to 12 weeks.[23] ACI has been found to have optimal outcomes in patients with lesions greater than 3 to 4 cm^2 without involvement of subchondral bone, young patients with greater than 2.5 cm^2 defects with high activity levels without involvement of subchondral bone, as well as some patients with large-diameter cartilage and subchondral bone defects.[24] Studies have found that 76% of patients treated with ACI were deemed to have successful treatment at 3-year follow-up,[25] and 71% of patients rated their outcomes as "good" or "excellent."[26] MACI is also known as third-generation ACI and was developed in an effort to improve traditional ACI technique outcomes while reducing complications.[27] In this technique, cultured autochondrocytes, as described above, are seeded onto a collagen bilayer matrix before implantation.[28,29] Zheng and colleagues[27] showed that in vitro MACI-regenerated cartilage-like tissue showed 75% hyaline-like cartilage. Ventura and colleagues[30] found that at 2-year follow-up 88% patients showed complete integration with surrounding endogenous cartilage on MRI. Second look arthroscopy and biopsy were performed in 6 patients and revealed full integration with surrounding cartilage as well as hyaline-like repair cartilage with type II cartilage. Augmentation with a collagen bilayer significantly improved cartilage regeneration in MACI, suggesting augmentation with biologics could further improve patient outcomes.

Osteochondral autografts and allografts are used to restore the natural architecture of the joint.[9] Autografts are used in patients with full-thickness osteochondral lesions less than 2.5 cm^2 as well as treatment of patients who have already failed previous cartilage restoration.[31,32] For lesions larger than 4 cm^2, osteochondral allograft (OCA) is often the procedure of choice. Although Frank and colleagues[33] found significant improvement in outcome scores at 5-year follow-up after OCA, a 32% reoperation rate was also noted. Levy and colleagues[34] found a reoperation rate of 47% by 10 years. In addition, 24% of knees had failed at a mean of 7.2 years. Predictors of allograft failure included 2 or more previous surgeries on the knee as well as age greater than 30 at the time of the operation.

Although these surgical treatments are effective for many patients, current research is focused on further improving outcome scores, reducing reoperation rates, and preventing the progression of these defects to OA through the use of biologics. The following sections describe how the senior author uses orthobiologics as an augmentation during the surgical management of focal chondral defects of the knee. Augmentation techniques, including BMAC, micronized allogeneic cartilage (MAC) matrix (BioCartilage), PRP, hyaluronic acid (HA), various scaffolds, growth factors, and cytokine modulation, have been described.

BONE MARROW ASPIRATE CONCENTRATE

The use of MSCs is currently being studied in many areas of orthopedics due to their regenerative potential. MSCs are able to be harvested from multiple sources, including bone marrow. Importantly, MSCs account for only 0.001% to 0.01% of nucleated cells in bone marrow.[35] Because of this, bone marrow aspirate can be harvested and processed via centrifuge to produce a more concentrated specimen. BMAC can then be used as a primary treatment or as adjunct to cartilage restoration surgery (Fig. 1). The utilization of BMAC stems from its extensive list of growth factors and cytokines, such as vascular endothelial growth factor, platelet-derived growth factor, transforming growth factor-beta (TGF-β), and bone morphogenetic proteins (BMP) -2 and -7, all of which are present in higher quantities when compared with other biologic products such as platelet-rich plasma (PRP).[36,37] In

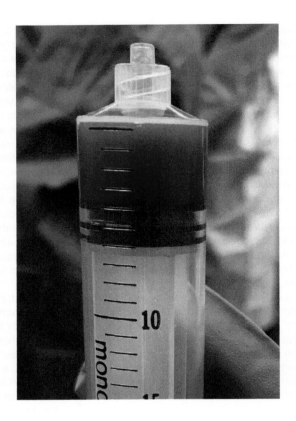

Fig. 1. BMAC.

addition, BMAC contains growth factors that are linked to chondrocyte proliferation, MSC differentiation, wound healing, and the suppression of proinflammatory cytokines.[38]

Early literature has been supportive of the use of BMAC as an adjunct to surgery for focal chondral defects. Saw and colleagues[39] augmented subchondral drilling with HA or BMAC + HA injections in a caprine model and found that at 24 weeks the BMAC + HA group's cartilage repair tissue was determined to have a significantly more hyaline-line structure as determined by the Gill score. Fortier and colleagues[40] used an equine model to compare microfracture augmented with BMAC and thrombin compared with microfracture alone in full-thickness, 15-mm defects and found that the BMAC group had significantly better International Cartilage Restoration Society (ICRS) scores with higher-quality repair tissue, increased type II collagen, and improved integration.

BMAC has also been studied as an adjunct to scaffolds. Enea and colleagues[41] studied 9 patients in whom microfracture was supplemented with a collagen membrane soaked in BMAC as treatment of focal chondral lesions. The study found that at 1-year follow-up, of the 4 patients who underwent second-look arthroscopy and cartilage biopsy, hyaline-like cartilage was seen in one patient, a mixture of hyaline-like cartilage and fibrocartilage was seen in 2 patients, and fibrocartilage alone was seen in one patient, suggesting BMAC is a safe and effective adjunct treatment in creating a more hyaline-like cartilage repair tissue. In addition, Krych and colleagues[42] showed that in patients with grade III or IV chondral lesions treated with a scaffold supplemented with BMAC, there was improved cartilage maturation and cartilage fill with mean quantitative T2 values closer to that of natural hyaline cartilage as compared with scaffold alone. Gobbi and colleagues[43] evaluated BMAC in combination with a collagen I/III matrix in focal cartilage defects with an average size of 8.3 cm and found a significant improvement in Tegner, Marx, Lysholm, VAS, IKDC subjective, and KOOS scores at 1, 2, and 3 years. The study also found complete filling of the defects on MRI in 80% of patients and less than 50% filling in 20% patients with complete integration of cartilage in 88% of patients. Gigante and colleagues[44] studied a 37-year-old man with a cartilage lesion on his medial femoral condyle treated with microfracture, BMAC, and a scaffold. The case report found the patient's MRI at 12 months showed substantial defect filling with tissue signal similar to that of surrounding tissue, and the patient remained asymptomatic throughout the 2-year follow-up.

In a study comparing BMAC in an HA scaffold (BMAC-HA) versus microfracture for full-thickness chondral defects, Gobbi and Whyte[45,46] found that all 50 patients significantly improved in IKDC scores, Lysholm, and Tegner at 2-year follow-up. In the microfracture group at 2-year follow-up, 64% of patients classified their functionality as "normal" and "nearly normal," whereas 100% of the BMAC-HA group classified their functionality as such. At 5-year follow-up, there was a significant decrease in the microfracture group, to 28%, in patients classifying their functionality as "normal" or "near normal," whereas the BMAC-HA group maintained their improvement across IKDC score, Lysholm, and Tegner.

In a prospective study, Gobbi and colleagues[47] compared MACI to the use of BMAC supplemented scaffolds in patellofemoral chondral lesions with a minimum follow-up of 3 years with average lesion sizes of 7.12 cm^2 and 5.54 cm^2, respectively. Both groups showed statistically significant improvements in IKDC score, KOOS score, VAS score, and Tegner. There was no significant difference between the improvements when both groups were compared with each other, except for IKDC scores, in which the BMAC group improved significantly more than the MACI patients.

Interestingly, Haleem and colleagues[48] studied expanded BMAC transplanted onto platelet-rich fibrin glue in 5 patients with full-thickness articular cartilage defects on either the lateral or the medial femoral condyle. Utilizing expanded BMAC involved a 2-step procedure as the MSCs underwent culture expansion for 2 weeks. All 5 of the patients experienced significant improvement in Lysholm and Revised Hospital for Special Surgery Knee Score at both 6 months and 1 year. MRI was completed at 1 year and showed complete defect fill with good integration of the repair tissue in 3 of the 5 patients. On second look arthroscopy at 1 year, one patient received an ICRS score of 11/12, denoting nearly normal cartilage.

Oladeji and colleagues[49] completed a cohort study to evaluate the effect of BMAC on integration of femoral condyle OCAs. In order to study this, grafts were saturated in BMAC for a minimum of 2 minutes before implantation (compared with no BMAC). Graft incorporation, as determined on radiographs, was significantly increased in the BMAC group at 6 weeks, 3 months, and 6 months. The BMAC group also showed significantly less sclerosis at 6 weeks and 3 months.

Taken together, these studies demonstrate that BMAC augmentation appears to play a role in regenerating a more hyaline-like repair tissue, improving patient-reported outcomes and improving radiographic evidence of healing. In addition, no major adverse events have been reported in these studies, suggesting that BMAC is a safe and efficacious adjunct treatment in cartilage defects.

MICRONIZED ALLOGRAFT ARTICULAR CARTILAGE AND PLATELET-RICH PLASMA

Another biologic option for patients with focal chondral defects involves the combination of particulated (or micronized) allograft articular cartilage with PRP. This technique is used most often as an augment to microfracture in an effort to form a more durable, hyaline-like cartilage rather than fibrocartilage.[21,50,51] BioCartilage Extracellular Matrix (Arthrex Inc, Naples, FL, USA) is one such product that is developed from allograft cartilage and contains the extracullular matrix that is found in normal articular cartilage. The application of BioCartilage and PRP can be done in a one-stage procedure unlike ACI. After preparation of the defect bed, typically using marrow stimulation techniques, the BioCartilage and PRP mixture is placed into the lesion and is then covered with a fibrin glue sealant to help it incorporate into surrounding cartilage and prevent expulsion.[50,51] In a study by Fortier and colleagues,[52] BioCartilage was used to fill 10-mm full-thickness cartilage defects at the trochlear ridge after microfracture in an equine model. The ICRS Score was significantly better in the BioCartilage augmentation group when compared with microfracture alone, as was the T2 relaxation time on MRI. Although there are multiple technique articles illustrating the implantation of BioCartilage in the knee, shoulder, and elbow[53] after microfracture, unfortunately, there is a paucity of data with regard to treatment outcomes of microfracture augmented with micronized allograft articular cartilage and PRP. Although future studies are required to determine if this technique is able to improve cartilage repair in vivo as well as to determine if it is able to provide patients with long-term pain relief, preliminary results suggest it is a safe and effective treatment for improving cartilage restoration techniques.

Notably, because these studies discuss the application of PRP in conjunction with BioCartilage, it is difficult to determine if the results are from the PRP or the MAC. PRP has shown promising results in vitro and in vivo for knee OA,[2,54–56] but its use is much less prevalent in the treatment of focal osteochondral defects, and results thus far have been mixed. Milano and colleagues[57] evaluated PRP in an ovine model as an adjunct to microfracture in the treatment of 8-mm^2 full-thickness chondral defects. The study compared microfracture alone, microfracture with PRP and fibrin placed within the microfracture holes, and an intra-articular injection of PRP after closure. At 6 months, the PRP + fibrin glue group showed well-integrated hyaline-like repair tissue that completely covered the defect, whereas the microfracture-alone group revealed continued exposure of subchondral bone with thin repair cartilage partially covering the defect. In the PRP injection group, repair tissue covered almost the entire defect. Although microfracture holes were no longer evident and cartilage repair tissue did have good integration with the surrounding tissue, it was thin and irregular in the central aspect of the defect. Smyth and colleagues[58] evaluated the use of leukocyte-rich PRP as an intra-articular injection in a rabbit model immediately after creating 3-mm^2 focal chondral defects in bilateral femoral condyles. In each rabbit, one defect was randomized to receive PRP and the other to receive saline. This study found that mean ICRS macroscopic score of the donor site was greater in the PRP-treated knees but did not reach statistical significance. However, microscopic assessment of the defect suggested increased tissue regeneration in the PRP group with greater glycosaminoglycan deposition and more type II collagen immunoreactivity throughout the repair tissue.

Van Bergen and colleagues[59] used a caprine model to analyze the use of PRP in adjunct to a demineralized bone matrix for the treatment of a 6-mm^2 osteochondral defect in the ankle. After 24 weeks, all of the defects were covered with fibrocartilage, and no significant differences were noted between the demineralized bone matrix group versus the adjunctive PRP group with regard to bone volume fraction, macroscopy, histomorphology, or fluorescent microscopy. Sun and colleagues[60] studied the effect of PRP as adjunctive treatment to polylactic glycolic carrier (PLGA) versus PLGA alone on 5-mm^2 osteochondral defects in a rabbit model. This study found that the group with the addition of PRP showed improved cartilage regeneration and integration of the hyaline-like cartilage. In a separate trial, Smyth and colleagues[61] analyzed the effect of PRP on the bony integration of osteochondral autografts in a rabbit model. The autografts were soaked in either PRP or saline for 10 minutes before implantation in the 2.7-mm^2 defect. The mean modified ICRS histologic score was significantly higher for the PRP group as compared with the control group. In addition, the mean score for graft integration was significantly higher in the PRP group as compared with the control group. As in the previous study, there was also an increase in glycosaminoglycan content and type II collagen immunoreactivity in the PRP group.

As stated above, PRP has shown promising results in the treatment of knee OA, suggesting it may have a similar effect in osteochondral defects. There is currently no standardized preparation technique for PRP, which has led to different concentrations of leukocytes and other factors in the final PRP preparation and may be the reason for conflicting results in numerous studies.[54,62–65] Studies have shown that higher concentrations of leukocytes are correlated with higher concentrations of proinflammatory molecules and that leukocyte-poor PRP is associated with improved bone marrow MSC proliferation, improved chondrogenesis, and decreased synoviocyte death.[66,67] The senior author's preferred technique of preparation of leukocyte-poor PRP is as follows. Venous blood is drawn from the patient, and the sample is centrifuged at 1500 rpm for 7 minutes. Centrifuge separates the sample into a bottom layer of red blood cells, an intermediate buffy layer filled with leukocytes and platelets, and a top layer of plasma (**Fig. 2**). This system uses a double syringe system (Arthrex Inc) so that after the initial centrifuge, the second syringe within the outer syringe fills with only the top layer of PRP.

Growth Factors

The 2 main growth factors used in microfracture supplementation are BMP-4 and -7, members of the TGF-β superfamily, because they have been shown to induce bone and cartilage formation as well as regulate cell proliferation and differentiation.[68] BMP-7 is also known as osteogenic protein-1 and is found in normal articular cartilage. Klein-Nulend and colleagues[69,70] showed that BMP-7 stimulates differentiation of cartilage from perichondrium tissue, which suggests BMP-7 is an important factor in cartilage regeneration and restoration.

Kuo and colleagues[71] studied the effect of microfracture augmented with BMP-7 in rabbits with patellar groove articular cartilage full-thickness defects as compared with microfracture alone and BMP-7 alone. The study found that when compared with the control group without treatment, microfracture alone increased the quantity of repair tissue present and improved the surface smoothness of the repair tissue. BMP-7 alone was found to increase the amount of repair tissue as well; however, it did not increase the quality of the repair cartilage. When combined, microfracture and BMP-7 were found to further increase the quantity of cartilage repair tissue as well as quality of the cartilage repair tissue. The investigators hypothesized that BMP-7 is acting directly on the MSCs released by the microfracture procedure. Similarly, Zhang and colleagues[72] studied BMP-4 as adjunct treatment to microfracture and decalcified cortical bone matrix in full-thickness defects in the trochlear groove in rabbits. This study found that animals that underwent microfracture with a scaffold and BMP-4 supplementation exhibited hyaline articular cartilage at 6 weeks and complete repair

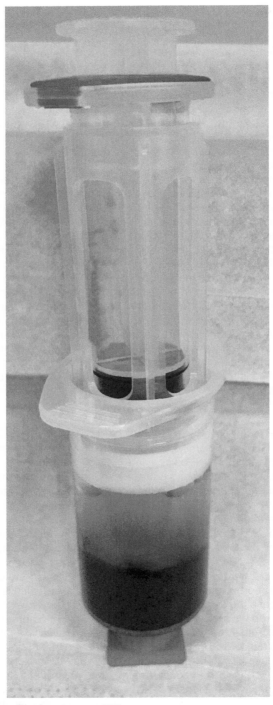

Fig. 2. Preparation of leukocyte-poor PRP.

of articular cartilage and subchondral bone at 12 weeks. In the microfracture-only group, the defects displayed concave fibrocartilage at 24 weeks, suggesting scaffold + BMP-4 improves regeneration of hyaline articular cartilage.

ADIPOSE-DERIVED MESENCHYMAL STEM CELLS

Another way MSCs can be derived is through adipose tissue, offering easy accessibility. Adipose-derived stem cells (ASCs) are obtained as lipoaspirate via liposuction. Next, the sample is purified and processed to isolate the ASCs via collagenase digestion, centrifugation, and culture. ASCs have anti-inflammatory effects and potential for regeneration of new cartilage in a defect. The senior author's preference is as follows: using the Lipogems technique (Lipogems International, Milan, Italy), the surgeon can harvest and process lipoaspirate intraoperatively, creating a single-step procedure with biologic adjunct. ASCs have been shown to have more stem cells per unit volume than BMAC,[73] and furthermore, have been shown have anti-inflammatory and chondroprotective effects intra-articularly.[74]

Bosetti and colleagues[75] analyzed ASC chondroinductive properties in vitro and showed that ASCs induce chondrocyte proliferation and extracelluar matrix production. The investigators demonstrated that microfragmented lipoaspirate clusters can give rise to spontaneous cell outgrowth in both floating culture conditions and in a 3-dimensional collagen matrix. Jo and colleagues[76] performed a randomized controlled trial and reported that intra-articular ASC injections resulted in a significant improvement in WOMAC scores at 6-month follow-up in patients with knee OA, a significant decrease in the size of the defect, and a significant increase in the amount of cartilage present in the joint. This study suggests ASCs would be a viable treatment option for focal cartilage defects because it would allow for a single-stage procedure for cartilage regeneration within the defect. However, more clinical data are needed to evaluate the safety and efficacy in vivo in treating these focal defects.

SUMMARY OF TREATMENT OPTIONS

There are many emerging options in the use of orthobiologics for the treatment of articular cartilage lesions. Although many studies show promising results of improvement in patient-reported outcomes as well as formation of a more hyaline-like cartilage repair tissue, additional high-level randomized controlled trials must be completed to further ensure safety, evaluate efficacy in different patient populations, and determine the appropriate protocol for preparation and administration of these biologics. There is no one treatment that is appropriate for each cartilage defect, but future research will help build a systematic algorithm based on the patient's defect size, age, activity level, and motivation to return to baseline in order to determine which biologic is the best fit.

REFERENCES

1. Filardo G, Kon E, DI Matteo B, et al. Leukocyte-poor PRP application for the treatment of knee osteoarthritis. Joints 2013;1(3):112–20.
2. Raeissadat SA, Rayegani SM, Hassanabadi H, et al. Knee osteoarthritis injection choices: Platelet-rich plasma (PRP) versus hyaluronic acid (A one-year randomized clinical trial). Clin Med Insights Arthritis Musculoskelet Disord 2015;8:1–8.
3. Gobbi A, Karnatzikos G, Mahajan V, et al. Platelet-rich plasma treatment in symptomatic patients with knee osteoarthritis: preliminary results in a group of active patients. Sports Health 2012;4(2):162–72.

4. Cole BJ, Karas V, Hussey K, et al. Hyaluronic acid versus platelet-rich plasma: a prospective, double-blind randomized controlled trial comparing clinical outcomes and effects on intra-articular biology for the treatment of knee osteoarthritis. Am J Sports Med 2017;45(2):339–46.

5. Hastie G, Soufi M, Wilson J, et al. Platelet rich plasma injections for lateral epicondylitis of the elbow reduce the need for surgical intervention. J Orthop 2018;15(1): 239–41.

6. Alessio-Mazzola M, Repetto I, Biti B, et al. Autologous US-guided PRP injection versus us-guided focal extracorporeal shock wave therapy for chronic lateral epicondylitis: a minimum of 2-year follow-up retrospective comparative study. J Orthop Surg 2018;26(1):1–8.

7. Roberts TT, Rosenbaum AJ. Bone grafts, bone substitutes and orthobiologics: the bridge between basic science and clinical advancements in fracture healing. Organogenesis 2012;8(4):114–24.

8. Ventura A, Terzaghi C, Legnani C, et al. Lateral ligament reconstruction with allograft in patients with severe chronic ankle instability. Arch Orthop Trauma Surg 2014;134:263–8.

9. Magnussen RA, Dunn WR, Carey JL, et al. Treatment of focal articular cartilage defects in the knee: a systematic review. Clin Orthop Relat Res 2008;466(4): 952–62.

10. McCormick F, Harris JD, Abrams GD, et al. Trends in the surgical treatment of articular cartilage lesions in the United States: an analysis of a large private-payer database over a period of 8 years. Arthroscopy 2014;30(2):222–6.

11. Wang KC, Waterman BR, Cotter EJ, et al. Fresh osteochondral allograft transplantation for focal chondral defect of the humerus associated with anchor arthropathy and failed SLAP repair. Arthrosc Tech 2017;6(4):e1443–9.

12. Chahal J, Gross AE, Gross C, et al. Outcomes of osteochondral allograft transplantation in the knee. Arthroscopy 2013;29(3):575–88.

13. Cole BJ, Farr J, Winalski CS, et al. Outcomes after a single-stage procedure for cell-based cartilage repair: a prospective clinical safety trial with 2-year follow-up. Am J Sports Med 2011;39(6):1170–9.

14. Widuchowski W, Widuchowski J, Trzaska T. Articular cartilage defects: Study of 25,124 knee arthroscopies. Knee 2007;14(3):177–82.

15. Curl WW, Krome J, Gordon ES, et al. Cartilage injuries: a review of 31,516 knee arthroscopies. Arthroscopy 1997;13(4):456–60.

16. Frank RM, Van Thiel GS, Slabaugh MA, et al. Clinical outcomes after microfracture of the glenohumeral joint. Am J Sports Med 2010;38(4):772–81.

17. Prakash D, Learmonth D. Natural progression of osteochondral defect in the femoral condyle. Knee 2002;9(1):7–10.

18. Dillon CF, Rasch EK, Gu Q, et al. Prevalence of knee osteoarthritis in the united states: arthritis data from the third national health and nutrition examination survey 1991-94. J Rheumatol 2006;33(11):2271–9.

19. Guettler JH, Demetropoulos CK, Yang KH, et al. Osteochondral defects in the human knee: Influence of defect size on cartilage rim stress and load redistribution to surrounding cartilage. Am J Sports Med 2004;32(6):1451–8.

20. Cole BJ, Pascual-Garrido C, Grumet RC. Surgical management of articular cartilage defects in the knee. J Bone Joint Surg Am 2009;91(7):1778–90.

21. Saltzman BM, Leroux T, Cole BJ. Management and surgical options for articular defects in the shoulder. Clin Sports Med 2017;36(3):549–72.

22. Romeo AA, Cole BJ, Mazzocca AD, et al. Autologous chondrocyte repair of an articular defect in the humeral head. Arthroscopy 2002;18(8):925–9.

23. Brittberg M, Lindahl A, Nilsson A, et al. Treatment of deep cartilage defects in the knee with autologous chondrocyte transplantation. N Engl J Med 1994;331(14): 889–95.
24. Niemeyer P, Andereya S, Angele P, et al. Autologous chondrocyte implantation (ACI) for cartilage defects of the knee: a guideline by the working group "Clinical Tissue Regeneration" of the German Society of Orthopaedic Surgery and Traumatology (DGOU)]. Knee 2016;23:426–35.
25. Zaslav K, Cole B, Brewster R, et al. A prospective study of autologous chondrocyte implantation in patients with failed prior treatment for articular cartilage defect of the knee: Results of the study of the treatment of articular repair (STAR) clinical trial. Am J Sports Med 2009;37(1):42–55.
26. Minas T, Bryant T. The role of autologous chondrocyte implantation in the patellofemoral joint. Clin Orthop Relat Res 2005;436:30–9.
27. Zheng M-H, Willers C, Kirilak L, et al. Matrix-Induced Autologous Chondrocyte Implantation (MACI®): biological and histological assessment. Tissue Eng 2007;13(4):737–46.
28. Seidl AJ, Kraeutler MJ. Management of articular cartilage defects in the glenohumeral joint abstract. J Am Acad Orthop Surg 2018;26(11):e230–7.
29. Bartlett W, Skinner JA, Gooding CR, et al. Autologous chondrocyte implantation versus matrix-induced autologous chondrocyte implantation for osteochondral defects of the knee: a Prospective, Randomized Study. J Bone Jt Surg Br 2005;87(5):640–5.
30. Ventura A, Memeo A, Borgo E, et al. Repair of osteochondral lesions in the knee by chondrocyte implantation using the MACI® technique. Knee Surgery Sports Traumatol Arthrosc 2012;20(1):121–6.
31. Wang KC, Cotter EJ, Davey A, et al. A treatment approach for articular cartilage defects. J Clin Orthop 2016;1(1):10–6.
32. Bajaj S, Petrera MO, Cole BJ. Lower extremity-articular cartilage injuries. Orthopaedic 2010;1:18. Available at: http://www.briancolemd.com/wp-content/themes/ypo-theme/pdf/cartilage-injury-and-treatment-2010-overview.pdf.
33. Frank RM, Lee S, Levy D, et al. Osteochondral allograft transplantation of the knee: analysis of failures at 5 years. Am J Sports Med 2017;45(4):864–74.
34. Levy YD, Görtz S, Pulido PA, et al. Do fresh osteochondral allografts successfully treat femoral condyle lesions? Clin Orthop Relat Res 2013;471(1):231–7.
35. Kasten P, Beyen I, Egermann M, et al. Instant stem cell therapy: characterization and concentration of human mesenchymal stem cells in vitro. Eur Cell Mater 2008;16:47–55.
36. Chahla J, Dean CS, Moatshe G, et al. Concentrated bone marrow aspirate for the treatment of chondral injuries and osteoarthritis of the knee: a systematic review of outcomes. Orthop J Sport Med 2016;4(1):1–8.
37. Holton J, Imam M, Ward J, et al. The basic science of bone marrow aspirate concentrate in chondral injuries. Orthop Rev (pavia) 2016;8(3):80–4.
38. Cotter EJ, Wang KC, Yanke AB, et al. Bone marrow aspirate concentrate for cartilage defects of the knee: from bench to bedside evidence. Cartilage 2018;9(2): 161–70.
39. Saw KY, Hussin P, Loke SC, et al. Articular cartilage regeneration with autologous marrow aspirate and hyaluronic acid: an experimental study in a goat model. Arthroscopy 2009;25(12):1391–400.
40. Fortier LA, Potter HG, Rickey EJ, et al. Concentrated bone marrow aspirate improves full-thickness cartilage repair compared with microfracture in the equine model. J Bone Joint Surg Am 2010;92(10):1927–37.

41. Enea D, Cecconi S, Calcagno S, et al. One-step cartilage repair in the knee: Collagen-covered microfracture and autologous bone marrow concentrate. A pilot study. Knee 2015;22(1):30–5.

42. Krych AJ, Nawabi DH, Farshad-Amacker NA, et al. Bone marrow concentrate improves early cartilage phase maturation of a scaffold plug in the knee. Am J Sports Med 2016;44(1):91–8.

43. Gobbi A, Karnatzikos G, Sankineani SR. One-step surgery with multipotent stem cells for the treatment of large full-thickness chondral defects of the knee. Am J Sports Med 2014;42(3):648–57.

44. Gigante A, Cecconi S, Calcagno S, et al. Arthroscopic knee cartilage repair with covered microfracture and bone marrow concentrate. Arthrosc Tech 2012;1(2):e175–80.

45. Whyte GP, Gobbi A, Sadlik B. Dry arthroscopic single-stage cartilage repair of the knee using a hyaluronic acid-based scaffold with activated bone marrow-derived mesenchymal stem cells. Arthrosc Tech 2016;5(4):e913–8.

46. Gobbi A, Whyte GP. One-stage cartilage repair using a hyaluronic acid-based scaffold with activated bone marrow-derived mesenchymal stem cells compared with microfracture. Am J Sports Med 2016;44(11):2846–54.

47. Gobbi A, Chaurasia S, Karnatzikos G, et al. Matrix-induced autologous chondrocyte implantation versus multipotent stem cells for the treatment of large patellofemoral chondral lesions: a nonrandomized prospective trial. Cartilage 2015;6(2):82–97.

48. Haleem AM, El Singergy AA, Sabry D, et al. The clinical use of human culture-expanded autologous bone marrow mesenchymal stem cells transplanted on platelet-rich fibrin glue in the treatment of articular cartilage defects: a pilot study and preliminary results. Cartilage 2010;1(4):253–61.

49. Oladeji LO, Stannard JP, Cook CR, et al. Effects of autologous bone marrow aspirate concentrate on radiographic integration of femoral condylar osteochondral allografts. Am J Sports Med 2017;45(12):2797–803.

50. Shin JJ, Mellano C, Cvetanovich GL, et al. Treatment of glenoid chondral defect using micronized allogeneic cartilage matrix implantation. Arthrosc Tech 2014;3(4):e519–22.

51. Wang KC, Frank RM, Cotter EJ, et al. Arthroscopic management of isolated tibial plateau defect with microfracture and micronized allogeneic cartilage–platelet-rich plasma adjunct. Arthrosc Tech 2017;6(5):e1613–8.

52. Fortier LA, Chapman HS, Pownder SL, et al. BioCartilage improves cartilage repair compared with microfracture alone in an equine model of full-thickness cartilage loss. Am J Sports Med 2016;44(9):2366–74.

53. Caldwell PE, Auerbach B, Pearson SE. Arthroscopic treatment of capitellum osteochondritis dissecans with micronized allogeneic cartilage scaffold. Arthrosc Tech 2017;6(3):e815–20.

54. Riboh JC, Saltzman BM, Yanke AB, et al. Effect of leukocyte concentration on the efficacy of platelet-rich plasma in the treatment of knee osteoarthritis. Am J Sports Med 2016;44(3):792–800.

55. Rayegani SM, Raeissadat SA, Sanei Taheri M, et al. Does intra articular platelet rich plasma injection improve function, pain and quality of life in patients with osteoarthritis of the knee? A randomized clinical trial. Orthop Rev (pavia) 2014;6(3). https://doi.org/10.4081/or.2014.5405.

56. Smith PA. Intra-articular autologous conditioned plasma injections provide safe and efficacious treatment for knee osteoarthritis. Am J Sports Med 2015;44(4):884–91.

57. Milano G, Sanna Passino E, Deriu L, et al. The effect of platelet rich plasma combined with microfractures on the treatment of chondral defects: an experimental study in a sheep model. Osteoarthr Cartil 2010;18(7):971–80.
58. Smyth NA, Haleem AM, Ross KA, et al. Platelet-rich plasma may improve osteochondral donor site healing in a rabbit model. Cartilage 2016;7(1):104–11.
59. Van Bergen CJA, Kerkhoffs GMMJ, Özdemir M, et al. Demineralized bone matrix and platelet-rich plasma do not improve healing of osteochondral defects of the talus: an experimental goat study. Osteoarthr Cartil 2013;21(11):1746–54.
60. Sun Y, Feng Y, Zhang CQ, et al. The regenerative effect of platelet-rich plasma on healing in large osteochondral defects. Int Orthop 2010;34(4):589–97.
61. Smyth NA, Haleem AM, Murawski CD, et al. The effect of platelet-rich plasma on autologous osteochondral transplantation. J Bone Joint Surg Am 2013;95:2185–93.
62. Dohan Ehrenfest DM, Rasmusson L, Albrektsson T. Classification of platelet concentrates: from pure platelet-rich plasma (P-PRP) to leucocyte- and platelet-rich fibrin (L-PRF). Trends Biotechnol 2009;27(3):158–67.
63. Şirin DY, Yilmaz I, Isyar M, et al. Does leukocyte-poor or leukocyte-rich platelet-rich plasma applied with biopolymers have superiority to conventional platelet-rich plasma applications on chondrocyte proliferation? Eklem Hastalik Cerrahisi 2017;28(3):142–51.
64. Giusti I, Di Francesco M, D'Ascenzo S, et al. Leukocyte depletion does not affect the in vitro healing ability of platelet rich plasma. Exp Ther Med 2018;15(4):4029–38.
65. McCarrel TM, Minas T, Fortier LA. Optimization of leukocyte concentration in platelet-rich plasma for the treatment of tendinopathy. J Bone Joint Surg Am 2012;94(19):1–8.
66. Xu Z, Yin W, Zhang Y, et al. Comparative evaluation of leukocyte-and platelet-rich plasma and pure platelet-rich plasma for cartilage regeneration. Sci Rep 2017;7(April 2016):1–14.
67. Braun HJ, Kim HJ, Chu CR, et al. The effect of platelet-rich plasma formulations and blood products on human synoviocytes. Am J Sports Med 2014;42(5):1204–10.
68. Chubinskaya S, Merrihew C, Cs-Szabo G, et al. Human articular chondrocytes express osteogenic protein-1. J Histochem Cytochem 2000;48(2):239–50.
69. Klein-Nulend J, Semeins CM, Mulder JW, et al. Stimulation of cartilage differentiation by osteogenic protein-1 in cultures of human perichondrium. Tissue Eng 1998;4(3):305–13.
70. Klein-Nulend J, Louwerse RT, Heyligers IC, et al. Osteogenic protein (OP-1, BMP-7) stimulates cartilage differentiation of human and goat perichondrium tissue in vitro. J Biomed Mater Res 1998;40(4):614–20.
71. Kuo AC, Rodrigo JJ, Reddi AH, et al. Microfracture and bone morphogenetic protein 7 (BMP-7) synergistically stimulate articular cartilage repair. Osteoarthr Cartil 2006;14(11):1126–35.
72. Zhang X, Zheng Z, Liu P, et al. The synergistic effects of microfracture, perforated decalcified cortical bone matrix and adenovirus-bone morphogenetic protein-4 in cartilage defect repair. Biomaterials 2008;29(35):4616–29.
73. Kasir R, Vernekar VN, Laurencin CT. Regenerative engineering of cartilage using adipose-derived stem cells. Regen Eng Transl Med 2015;1(1–4):42–9.
74. Ter Huurne M, Schelbergen R, Blattes R, et al. Antiinflammatory and chondroprotective effects of intraarticular injection of adipose-derived stem cells in experimental osteoarthritis. Arthritis Rheum 2012;64(11):3604–13.

75. Bosetti M, Borrone A, Follenzi A, et al. Human lipoaspirate as autologous inject-able active scaffold for one-step repair of cartilage defects. Cell Transplant 2016; 25(6):1043–56.
76. Jo C, Lee Y, SHIN W. Intra-articular injection of mesenchymal stem cells for the treatment of osteoarthritis of the knee: a proof-of-concept clinical trial. Stem Cells 2014;32:1254–66.

Ortho-Biologics for Osteoarthritis

Kyla Huebner, MSc, MD, PhD[a], Rachel M. Frank, MD[b],
Alan Getgood, MPhil, MD, FRCS (Tr&Orth)[a],*

KEYWORDS

• PRP • Autologous conditioned serum • Stem cell • Bone marrow • Osteoarthritis

KEY POINTS

• This review seeks to shed light on the current literature in the use of key ortho-biologics and their potential use in the treatment of osteoarthritis.

• The literature supports the safety of viscosupplementation, platelet-rich plasma, autologous conditioned serum, bone marrow aspirate concentrate and adipose derived stromal cell therapy in the treatment of OA.

• The clinical efficacy of these treatments continues to be investigated in comparative studies and meta-analyses.

• Further work is still required to fully understand the clinical role for orthobiologics in OA treatment.

INTRODUCTION

Osteoarthritis (OA) is a debilitating disease affecting approximately 27 million Americans.[1] The most common symptoms of OA are pain and physical limitations that have a significant effect on people's quality of life and their social and economic activities.[2,3] Because of the increasing life expectancy, increasing numbers of elderly, and increasing prevalence of obesity in North America, the prevalence of OA will continue to increase. There are currently limited options for treatment and prevention of OA, with joint replacement often the ultimate outcome. The cost of joint replacements is around $55,000 per person with complication rates of approximately 1% to 10% and mortality rates of 0.25%.[4] In order to reduce costs to the medical system and the risks and costs to patients, we need a better understanding of the disease pathophysiology, improved early detection, and strategies for disease prevention and early disease management. Ortho-biologics may be one such option for the treatment of OA.

Disclosure Statement: None.
[a] Division of Orthopaedic Surgery, Western University, Fowler Kennedy Sports Medicine Clinic, 3M Centre, 1151 Richmond Street, London, Ontario N6A 3K7, Canada; [b] University of Colorado, Boulder, CO, USA
* Corresponding author.
E-mail address: agetgoo@uwo.ca

Clin Sports Med 38 (2019) 123–141
https://doi.org/10.1016/j.csm.2018.09.002

Ortho-biologics as defined by the American Academy of Orthopaedic Surgeons (AAOS) are biological substances found naturally in the body that help injuries heal more quickly.[5] These substances include any biologically derived conductive material that aids in repair and regeneration of bone, muscle, tendons, ligaments and cartilage. There are many treatments that now fit under this overarching term. These treatments include platelet-rich plasma (PRP), prolotherapy, ozone therapy, autologous conditioned serum (ACS), bone marrow aspirate concentrates (BMACs), adipocyte-derived stem cells, mesenchymal-derived concentrates, amniotic-derived cell concentrates, cord blood–derived cell concentrates, interleukin therapies, and alpha-2 macrophages. For the purpose of this review, the authors focus on viscosupplementation, PRP, ACS, BMACs, and other cell-derived therapies, as these are currently in clinical use.

VISCOSUPPLEMENTATION

Viscosupplementation consists of hyaluronic acid (HA) treatments injected into the joint for pain relief and possible antiinflammatory effect.[6] HA is an anionic, nonsulfated glycosaminoglycan found in connective tissues, epithelium, and neural tissue. It is formed in the plasma membrane and is one of the main components of the extracellular matrix, contributing to cell proliferation and migration. HA is found within joints providing viscoelastic properties to the synovial fluid. In OA, there is a reduction in HA synthesis with increased HA degradation, in turn, leading to a lower molecular weight in the synovium, synovial fluid, and cartilage.[7] HA therapy provides relief via various pathways, including suppression of proinflammatory cytokines and chemokines through the synthesis of antiinflammatory mediators.[8] In a systematic review by Altman and colleagues, 48 articles were analyzed to evaluate the antiinflammatory effect of HA in OA.[9] They found that proinflammatory cytokines (interleukin 1β [IL-1β]), tumor necrosis factor α (TNFα), and interferon γ can regulate HA synthase expression. HA binds to cell surface receptors, such as CD44, toll-like receptor (TLR) 2 and 4, layilin, and intracellular adhesion molecule-1 (ICAM-1). In binding to CD44, it suppresses proinflammatory cytokines, matrix metalloproteinases (MMPs), proteoglycans, and prostaglandin E_2 synthesis via CD44 through the downregulation of nuclear factor (NF)-κB. HA also activates the innate immune response via TLR-2. HA treatment was shown to bind to TLR-2 and TLR-4 and decrease TNFα, IL-1β, IL-17, MMP13, and inducible nitric oxide. Layilin is expressed in human articular chondrocytes and synoviocytes; by binding to layilin HA suppressed the expression of IL-1β and MMP1 and 13. ICAM-1 activates the NF-κB regulatory system activating proinflammatory cytokines; HA binds to ICAM-1 and inhibits its action thereby preventing inflammation.[9,10]

Early studies of HA treatments in OA had mixed results. In a large meta-analysis of 89 trials containing 12,667 participants, 71 studies showed a modest effect in decreasing pain, whereas the remainder showed no effect. Fourteen studies had significant adverse effects related to HA injections. Rutjes and colleagues[11] concluded based on these early studies that HA therapy had a clinically irrelevant benefit with significant adverse reactions.

Miller and Block[12] did 2 meta-analyses evaluating 26 articles with a total of 4866 subjects for the safety and efficacy of HA. They found that there was a large treatment effect for up to 26 weeks for pain relief and improved Western Ontario and McMaster Universities Osteoarthritis Index (WOMAC) scores. There were no significant adverse effects reported in this series of studies.[13] In another meta-analysis of high-quality level 1 randomized controlled trials (RCTs), 12 studies consisting of 1794 participants were analyzed. Early on, between 1 and 3 months, corticosteroid injections had improved outcomes in the WOMAC score and lower visual analog scale (VAS) scores. However, at 6 months, the effect of HA was better than corticosteroids in OA.[14] In another study of 13 articles, HA was shown to have greater effects up to 1 year compared with nonsteroidal antiinflammatories and corticosteroids.[15] Bhandari and colleagues[16] reviewed 8 meta-analyses and found that by 26 weeks there were significant improvements in pain, functional scores, and stiffness after HA injections in patients with mild to moderate OA. In addition, they found HA to be well tolerated and safe. Importantly, they observed that HAs with a molecular weight greater than 6000 kDA or greater had the greatest treatment effect on pain at 13 weeks and *3000 kDA or greater has the greatest treatment effect on pain at 26 weeks*. In addition to one-time injections, patients often require multiple treatments. A meta-analysis of 7404 patients showed that repeat HA injections were safe in patients with OA. In 95% of patients who had an adverse event, it was at the time of the first treatment; there was no increase in frequency or severity of adverse events with repeat treatments. The adverse event rate was 0.008 with repeat injections.[17]

In light of the mixed results in the literature and the changes in AAOS guidelines, a US and a European consensus were formed to help guide the use of HA in OA. The European Viscosupplementation Consensus Group determined that, based on an extensive review of the literature, if HA injections were successful previously, a repeat attempt at treatment should be undertaken. They also recommended the use of HA injections in young patients at high risk of progression of OA and competitive athletes in a possible attempt to slow the progression of OA.[18] A similar US task force of rheumatologists, orthopedic surgeons, physiatrists, sports medicine physicians, and nurses was formed to study HA injections in OA. They reviewed 100 studies that suggested HA was superior to placebo treatments. Based on these studies, they came up with 8 various clinical scenarios by which to use HA injections (3 appropriate uses and 5 unclear uses)[19] (**Table 1**).

Table 1	
Clinical scenarios for the use of HA listed by Bhadra and colleagues	
1. Symptomatic adults with mild or moderate OA of the knee who have clinically and radiologically confirmed disease who have not received other therapies for the knee	Appropriate
2. Symptomatic adults with severe mild or moderate OA of the knee who have clinically and radiologically confirmed disease and have failed other nonpharmacologic or pharmacologic therapies for the knee	Appropriate
3. Symptomatic adults with mild or moderate OA of the knee who have clinically and radiologically confirmed disease who have incomplete response to other therapies for the knee	Appropriate
4. Symptomatic adults with mild or moderate OA of the knee who are intolerant of, have a high-risk of adverse reaction to, or who are contraindicated for pharmacologic agents for the knee (oral, topical, or intra-articular)	Unclear
5. Symptomatic adults who have mechanical meniscus pathology with underlying OA of the knee	Unclear
6. Symptomatic adults with OA of the knee who have had a significant adverse reaction to an intra-articular HA product	Unclear
7. Symptomatic adults with OA of the knee who have active inflammatory arthritis (rheumatoid arthritis, gout, and so forth)	Unclear
8. Symptomatic adults with OA of the knee who have synovitis of the knee with significant effusion	Unclear

From Bhadra AK, Altman R, Dasa V, et al. Appropriate use criteria for hyaluronic acid in the treatment of knee osteoarthritis in the United States. Cartilage 2017;8(3):239; with permission.

In practice, HA is widely used as a part of the treatment algorithm for mild to moderate OA despite the lack of consensus and the current US and Canadian treatment guidelines. It likely has some benefit in certain patients and is worth a trial of treatment in those who are candidates.

PLATELET-RICH PLASMA

As cartilage is nonvascular, its nourishment is based on diffusion. Therefore, intra-articular injections at high concentrations are often the preferred method to aid in cartilage regeneration. PRP, which has a higher concentration of platelets than whole blood, has been an interesting option for use in OA. PRP is a natural concentrate of autologous factors obtained by centrifugation or filtration of the patients' blood. It is obtained at a low cost, simple to obtain, and minimally invasive. PRP is thought to work via biologically active proteins (including platelet-derived growth factor [PDGF], transforming growth factor [TGF], insulinlike growth factor, fibroblast growth factor, and vascular endothelial growth factor [VEGF][20]) expressed by platelets leading to gene expression by binding to transmembrane receptors in target cells. PDGF is a chemoattractant and stimulator of cell proliferation. TGF is a polypeptide that is abundant in platelets and bone and plays an important role in wound healing; it may negatively influence angiogenesis and promotes matrix production by fibroblasts and stimulates the production of VEGF. VEGF is a family of proteins that act through the kinase family expressed on endothelial cells, which stimulate blood vessel formation and exert a trophic effect on endothelial cells. VEGF is also proinflammatory and stimulates leukocyte adhesion to endothelial cells. As a result of these growth hormones, cellular recruitment, migration, growth, and morphogenesis are triggered and inflammation is decreased.[21] Therefore, it has been widely used and studied as a noninvasive treatment of cartilage regeneration in OA.

As PRP is an autologous product, there is a lot of variability within individual patients. Differences in patients' daily platelet levels, procurement methods, concentration mechanisms, and exogenous factors to enhance platelet activation can all contribute to varied PRP preparations. Platelet concentration varies significantly between procurement method and time of draw.[22,23] Platelet concentrates have been recorded as between 200×10^3 and 1000×10^3 platelets per microliter, with no consensus existing as to which concentration has the best outcomes. However, concentrations greater than this have been demonstrated to be biologically unfavorable.[23,24] In addition to the variation in draw times and platelet concentration, there can be variability in leukocytes within the RPR formulation. It is debatable whether leukocytes are beneficial or detrimental, as they have the potential to aid in healing; however, they can also be the cause of increased injury and adverse reactions.[24] Leukocytes adversely increase local inflammation, beneficially produce VEGF, have antimicrobial effects and are restorative to tissues.[25–27] The addition of leukocytes to PRP has also been shown to enhance the concentration of growth factors in PRP.[27] There are 2 different types of commercially available system for PRP: one producing a leukocyte-rich PRP (LR-PRP) and the other producing a leukocyte-poor PRP (LP-PRP). A buffy coat system, which uses a high centrifugation rate for a longer time, produces LR-PRP.[28] Plasma-based systems produce LP-PRP; it uses slower centrifugation or filtration for a shorter time.[28] The literature is still split on the benefit of LR-PRP versus LP-PRP for a given for a given clinical indication. Exogenous factors can also be added to PRP formulations, the most common being thrombin. Thrombin activates platelets and is often used in combination with calcium chloride.[22] Thrombin plus calcium chloride was shown to increase the release of growth factors in PRP, releasing 100% of growth factors by 1 hour.[29]

Preclinical studies have been supportive of the use of PRP for the regeneration of joint tissue in OA. PRP increases chondrocyte proliferation and increases the production of proteoglycans and type II collagen in vitro.[30–33] In animal models PRP leads to improved cartilage regeneration,[34] and enhances meniscal cells[35] and synoviocytes.[36] PRP has also been shown to have an antiinflammatory effect.[37,38] Based on these studies of the basic biology involved in PRP, there is evidence to support that PRP enhances cartilage repair and slows degradation.

The initial investigation into the use of PRP injections to treat OA was published in 2008. It was a retrospective observational study of 60 patients, which showed favorable outcomes after intra-articular PRP injections.[39] It was not until 2012 that the first RCT was published. To the authors' knowledge since then, 7 systematic reviews/meta-analyses have been published. This section summarizes the current clinic evidence for PRP in OA focusing on meta-analyses. **Table 2** shows a summary of these articles.

Chang and colleagues[40] in 2014 performed a systematic review and meta-analysis analyzing the effectiveness of PRP in treating chondral lesions in the knee. The investigators included 8 single-arm studies, 3 quasi-experimental studies, and 5 RCTs consisting of 1543 subjects. PRP showed efficacy for 12 months after injection and its effectiveness was better and more prolonged than HA injections in patients with mild-moderate OA.[40] A level 1 systematic review and meta-analysis performed by Laudy and colleagues[41] in 2014 compared PRP with HA and placebo. Six RCTs and 4 non-RCTs were included. They found improved functional outcomes of WOMAC, the VAS, and Lequesne index after PRP injections compared with HA and placebo.[41]

In another meta-analysis of PRP in OA, the use of LR-PRP and LP-PRP was investigated and clinical outcomes (WOMAC and International Knee Documentation Committee [IKDC]) and adverse effects were compared. They included 6 RCTs and 3 retrospective studies containing 1055 participants. LP-PRP had better WOMAC and IKDC scores than HA or controls, whereas there was no difference in LR-PRP scores. Both LP-PRP and LR-PRP had higher adverse reactions compared with HA and controls, being primarily swelling and pain.[42]

Meheux and colleagues[43] performed a systematic review of level 1 RCTs to determine whether PRP improves patient-reported outcomes at 6 and 12 months and to determine any differences between PRP or HA or placebo treatment at 6 and 12 months. After a quality assessment using the modified Coleman methodology score, 6 articles were analyzed. All but one study showed significant differences in clinical outcomes between groups for pain and function. Posttreatment PRP scores were significantly better than for HA at 3 and 6 months. In addition, PRP injections resulted in significant clinical improvements up to 12 months.[43] In another systematic review by Sadabad and colleagues[44] in 2016 evaluating 7 studies consisting of 722 participants, they found that PRP led to significantly improved WOMAC scores compared with HA.

In the most recent meta-analysis by Dai and colleagues,[45] 10 RCTs consisting of 1069 participants were used to compare PRP injections with HA at 6 and 12 months. At 6 months there was no difference in clinical outcomes between HA and PRP treatments; however, by 12 months PRP treatment resulted in significantly improved WOMAC, IKDC, and Lequesne scores.[45]

Overall the body of literature suggests that PRP is a promising therapy for symptom relief and improved functional outcomes in patients with OA for at least 12 months.

Table 2
Summary of meta-analyses looking at PRP

Study	Studies Included	Databases	Dates	Comparison	Sample Size	Average Follow-up	Outcome Measures	Results
Chang et al,[40] 2014	16 Studies • 8 single arm • 3 quasi-experimental • 5 RCTs	MEDLINE	2010–2013	PRP vs HA	1543	12 mo	IKDC KOOS WOMAC	PRP significantly improved scores more than HA. PRP was more effective in less severe OA.
Laudy et al,[41] 2014	10 Studies • 6 RCTs • 6 non-RCTs	MEDLINE Embase CINHAL Web of Science Cochrane database	2011–2013	PRP vs HA PRP vs placebo	1110	6 mo	WOMAC VAS Lequesne	PRP significantly improved scores than HA. PRP significantly improved scores more than placebo.
Riboh et al,[42] 2015	9 Studies • 6 RCTs • 3 prospective	MEDLINE Embase Cochrane database	2011–2013	LP PRP vs LR PRP	1055	Not reported	IKDC WOMAC Adverse reactions VAS Lequesne Tegner Marx KOOS SF-36 MRI	LP-PRP improved WOMAC scores compared with placebo. There were similar adverse events between LP-PRP and LR-PRP.

Study	No. of Studies	Databases	Years	Comparison	N	Follow-up	Outcomes	Results
Meheux et al,[43] 2016	6 Studies	PubMed, Cochrane database, Central register of controlled trials, Scopus, Sport discus	2011–2015	PRP vs HA	739	6–12 mo	WOMAC, IKDC, KOOS, VAS, Lequesne	PRP had improved outcomes compared with baseline greater than HA.
Sadabad et al,[44] 2016	6 Studies	PubMed, Cochrane database, Scopus, Void database	2005–2015	PRP vs HA	722	5–48 wk	WOMAC	PRP significantly improved WOMAC scores than HA.
Dai et al,[45] 2017	10 RCTs	PubMed, Embase, Scopus, Cochrane database	2011–2016	PRP vs HA, PRP vs saline	1069	3–12 mo	WOMAC, IKDC, Lequesne	At 6 mo, there was no difference between treatments. At 12 mo, PRP had improved outcomes compared with both HA and saline.

Abbreviations: CINHAL, Cumulative Index to Nursing and Allied Health Literature; IDKC, International Knee Documentation Committee; KOOS, Knee Injury and OA Outcome Score; SF-36, 36-Item Short-Form Health Survey.

LP-PRP provided better functional outcomes compared with placebo versus LR-PRP, whereas both have increased adverse events compared with HA or placebo. Further work needs to be done to determine if it has any disease-modifying effects.

AUTOLOGOUS CONDITIONED SERUM

Inflammation has been shown to play a key role in the pathophysiology of OA. Proinflammatory cytokines and MMPs are upregulated in the synovial fluid and tissue of patients with OA,[46] including significantly increased levels of IL-1 receptors on chondrocytes[47] and synovial fibroblasts.[48] IL-1 receptor antagonist (IL-1Ra) is a competitive receptor antagonist and natural inhibitor of IL-1, which blocks IL-1's signaling activity.[49] It was proposed as a therapeutic agent in the early 1980s.[50] Meijer and colleagues[51] created an ortho-biologic based on this known as ACS, marketed as Orthokine. ACS is a process by which venous blood is collected and rapid synthesis of IL-1Ra, IL-4, IL-10, and growth factors are stimulated with glass beads. Orthokine has been on the market since 1998 and has been used in both animal models and orthopedic patients. One proposed application is in patients with OA.

In a level 1 RCT by Baltzer and colleagues[52] in 2008, 376 participants were treated with ACS, HA, or placebo. Participants were followed for 26 weeks using an intention-to-treat analysis. Outcome measures including VAS, WOMAC, Short-Form 8, and the global patient assessment, were assessed at baseline, 7, 13, and 26 weeks. The ACS group had improved WOMAC, VAS, and Short-Form 8 scores compared with baseline and a larger improvement compared with the HA-treated group. At 2 years after treatment, outcomes persisted in the ACS group over the HA and placebo group.

Auw Yang and colleagues,[53] in a 30-month multicenter RCT, compared ACS with a saline control in decreasing symptoms of OA. One hundred sixty-seven participants were treated with either saline or ACS over 3 weeks. Participants completed the VAS, Knee Injury and OA Outcome Score (KOOS), the Knee Society Clinical Rating System, and the WOMAC scores at baseline, 3, 6, 9, and 12 months. Adverse events were similar between groups. The primary outcome measure of this study was not met. Both ACS and placebo-treated patients had a significant improvement in all measures. ACS resulted in a significant improvement in the KOOS score compared with placebo.

In observational studies by Baselga Garcia-Escudero and Miguel Hernandez Trillos[54] and Rutgers and colleagues,[55] ACS treatment was compared with placebo in patients with grade I to IV OA. Baselga Garcia-Escudero and Miguel Hernandez Trillos[54] found that of 118 patients who had ACS injections, there was a significant improvement at 24 months compared with baseline in pain and function scores. Whereas in Rutgers and colleagues'[55] smaller study of patients who self-selected their treatment, there was no difference between placebo and ACS.

In a more recent study looking at 100 patients treated with ACS and followed for a year, there was an 84% improvement in pain and satisfaction at 6 months and a 91% improvement at 12 months after treatment.[56] In a level 1 RCT published by Smith[57] in 2016, ACS proved to be effective for the treatment of OA in 30 patients. The study was designed as a feasibility study in which patients were randomized to receive either ACS or placebo. WOMAC scores were the primary outcome, and patients were followed for 1 year. There were no adverse effects from the ACS treatments. Furthermore, there was a significant increase in WOMAC scores at 1 year from baseline in the ACS-treated group (78% increase), whereas the placebo group had only a 7% increase from baseline. In a subsequent small trial by Zarringam and colleagues[58] examining the role of ACS to prevent surgery in the long-term, there was no difference in rates of surgery between patients treated with ACS versus those who were not.

There is some preliminary evidence supporting the use of ACS in the treatment of OA. Unfortunately, studies have yet to reproduce the cytokine changes seen in vitro in human studies[59]; clinical outcomes are varied across the literature.

BONE MARROW ASPIRATE CONCENTRATE

Cell-based therapies have emerged as a new potential therapeutic approach in musculoskeletal disease. OA is one of the prominent targets for these therapies. However, most are still in the proof-of-concept phase. BMACs are collected from bone marrow aspirates and processed immediately for use and have been one of the most popular sources for cell therapy. Bone aspiration is typically performed in a percutaneous fashion and is fast, safe, and associated with low donor site morbidity. Once collected, it is in a single-cell suspension that can be immediately processed and used with minimal manipulation,[60,61] therefore, not requiring significant clinical trials to gain regulatory approval. These preparations are classified through the US Food and Drug Administration (FDA) as a 361 product and, hence, are not subject to premarket review and approval, making it easy to access as a treatment. It is most commonly collected from the anterior iliac crest, but yields are higher from the posterior iliac crest.[62] Other areas for harvest include, but are not limited to, the proximal tibia, the proximal humerus, and intercondylar notch. The techniques by which bone marrow aspirates are collected and processed have a large effect on the number of nucleated cells. It is key to maintain low aspiration volumes, because bone marrow–derived cells are collected in the first 2 mL of the aspirate and after that are diluted by the blood volume.[63]

BMAC is rich in mesenchymal stem cells (MSCs), which play a key role in cartilage regeneration. MSCs have a potential for self-renewal and multipotency toward cells of the mesodermal lineage. They have reparative, homing, and trophic properties causing them to migrate to areas of damage; once at the site of injury, they release numerous factors, including many that help in healing.[64] In addition to MSCs, BMAC has recently been shown to have an increased concentration of IL-1Ra protein, which, in combination with the other constituents, may provide antiinflammatory and immunomodulatory effects.[65]

In a prospective case series by Wakitani and colleagues,[66] 24 patients underwent a high tibial osteotomy along with BMAC cell transplantation. Their knees were evaluated arthroscopically at 42 weeks after treatment, and all regions of cartilage defects were found to be covered in a white metachromatic tissue. Further histologic and arthroscopic grades showed a significant improvement compared with baseline. However, there were no differences in clinical outcomes. Further studies by Koh and colleagues[67] were less successful at demonstrating normal coverage with a second-look arthroscopy. In a retrospective case series of 37 patients who had BMAC treatment, patients were found to have higher IKDC and Tegner activity scale scores at 2 years and a 94% satisfaction rate. However, they demonstrated at 2 years that 76% of cartilage defects were still abnormal or severely abnormal. Jo and colleagues[68] in 2014 were able to demonstrate in a small pilot phase I and II study that BMAC was safe and improved WOMAC scores at 6 months in patients treated with high-dose cell numbers (1×10^8). On arthroscopic evaluation there was a hyline like cap and histologic and arthroscopic scores were higher than pretreatment and compared with the low-dose cell treatment.

Multiple small studies have demonstrated improved clinical outcomes after BMAC treatment. In a 6-patient series there were no adverse events by 1 year; by 6 months participants had improved pain and were able to walk further. In addition, T2 relaxation MRIs demonstrated increased cartilage thickness at 6 months compared with pre-treatment MRIs.[69] Similarly, Orozco and colleagues[70] found increased cartilage on MRI over areas of previous poor cartilage coverage at 1 year (n = 12). In a further study, 75 patients also had improved VAS, WOMAC, and Lequesne scores. BMAC therapy improved VAS, IKDC, Short-Form 36, KOOS, and Lysholm in mild to moderate (grade I–III) OA, whereas there was no change in participants with severe grade IV OA.[71] BMAC treatment was also found to be safe in a single blinded pilot RCT after 6 months of treatment, with VAS scores improved from baseline but no different compared with saline controls.[72] Sampson and colleagues[73] found when BMAC was given in conjunction with PRP in a case series of 125 participants followed for 8 weeks that there was an absolute reduction in pain and a 91.7% satisfaction rate. Furthermore, in a comparison of BMAC with placebo to PRP injections, there were low rates of adverse events and improved lower extremity functional scale (LEFS) and pain scores compared with baseline and placebo and PRP in 615 patients.[74]

Lastly, in 2015, Centeno and Bashir[75] examined registry data of 373 patients treated with a low-cell-count ($\leq 4 \times 10^8$) or high-cell-count ($>4 \times 10^8$) BMAC. At 12 months, both low- and high-cell-count treatment groups had better outcomes (IKDC, LEFS, and pain scores) compared with baseline. The higher-cell-count treated group also had significantly lower pain scores than the low-cell-count group.[75]

Despite the high volume of BMAC used clinically, there is a very low level of evidence to support its use. Further and more methodologically stringent studies need to be done in order to evaluate the benefit of BMAC for the treatment of OA.

ADIPOSE-DERIVED STROMAL CELL THERAPY

Adipose-derived stromal cell therapy, also known as adipose stromal vascular (ASC) fraction, has gained recent popularity as a treatment that falls under the 361 product as a minimally manipulated product. ASC is collected and isolated in a closed disposable system. It is most commonly collected from lipo-aspiration of the abdomen but can also be collected from the fat pad in the knee. Once collected, the ASC is processed in cylinders with beads and is filtered and injected into the patients' joints.[76] This process can be done in a single outpatient procedure making it desirable from a patient perspective. ASC contains a high frequency of adipose-derived stem cells; however, the frequency of stem cells relative to mononuclear cells varies significantly.[77]

Initial basic science studies have been performed in vitro. For example, in one study, chondrocytes from OA patient donors were cocultured with ASC. Maumus and colleagues[78] found no effect on chondrocyte proliferation but did note a decrease in apoptosis. ASC treatment decreased TGFβ secretion by chondrocytes and led to the induction of human growth factor (HGF), which was reversed with anti-HGF treatment. IL-1, TNFα, tissue inhibitor of metalloproteinase 1 and 2, and MMP1 and 9 were not changed by ASC treatment.[78] Further studies compared chondrocytes with synoviocytes cocultured with abdominal fat, Hoffa fat pad, or subcutaneous hip fat.[67,79–81] There was no difference between the sources of ASC; all decreased levels of IL-1, TNFα, IL-6, CXCL1, CXCL8, CCL3, and CCL5. This reduction was conditional on the chondrocytes and synoviocytes producing high levels of inflammatory factors. Furthermore, they demonstrated that these decreases were due to alterations in the prostaglandin E_2 and cyclooxygenase 2 pathways.[82] Jin and colleagues,[79] in 2017, harvested chondrocytes from patients with and without OA undergoing abdominal surgery and treated the chondrocytes with ASC from lipoaspiration. Chondrocytes from OA donors had decreased miR-373, which mediated an increase in P2X76, both involved in inflammation. When chondrocytes were stimulated with IL-1β, secretion of inflammatory factors increased; this was suppressed by the addition of ASC.

Preclinical animal studies have shown some promising results following ASC therapy. New Zealand white rabbits induced with OA were treated with either saline or ASC injection collected from the infrapatellar fat pad 12 weeks after induction.[83] By 20 weeks, radiographic images showed that rabbits had developed OA and that ASC decreased the amount of joint space narrowing, subchondral sclerosis, and osteophytes. The cartilage also showed less signs of degeneration by gross and histologic examination after ASC injection.[83] When ASC was injected into rabbits with OA and healthy rabbits, there were no adverse effects; both the OA rabbits and healthy rabbits had preserved cartilage on MRI, radiograph, and histopathology.[84] Parrilli and colleagues[85] compared dosages of ASC (2×10^6 vs 6×10^6) injected into the rabbit knee joint with OA. They found increased bone turnover and cartilage repair in both groups.

Adipose stem cells harvested from rats maintained fibroblast morphology and differentiated into chondrocytes and stimulated cartilage regeneration when injected into the knees of OA rats.[86] Mei and colleagues[87] demonstrated that ASC therapy versus placebo in a rat model of OA decreased cartilage degeneration seen grossly and histologically by 8 to 12 weeks after treatment. When xanthan gum was added to the ASC injection, there were improved results compared with ASC alone as well as a decrease in IL-1β, TNFα, and MMP3 and 13.[88] In culture, chondrocytes exposed to subcutaneous ASC had increased levels of IL-10[87] and improved chondrogenesis and immunosuppression.[89] ACS was also shown to increase proteoglycan production in mice.[90]

In phase I clinical trials of ASC therapy in knee OA, dose-escalation treatments were all found to be safe, with adverse effects consisting of swelling and pain that were limited to 24 hours after injection. At the low dose, ASC therapy improved WOMAC scores as well.[91] Similarly, Russo and colleagues[92] found ASC therapy was safe in a trial of 30 participants and had a greater than 10-point improvement in all clinical outcomes (KOOS, IKDC, Lysholm, Tegner, and VAS) by 12 months. In a small study of 6 patients, there were no infections after treatment, C-reactive protein remained at baseline levels, and patients had improved range of motion and timed up-and-go at 3 months after treatment, and improved WOMAC and VAS scores for up to a year after treatment.[93] Bansal and colleagues[81] showed favorable results of ASC treatment in mild grade I to II OA. Ten patients with OA undergoing liposuction were treated with ASC and had improvements in WOMAC and 6-minute walk distance up to 2 years after treatment. Six patients also had a 0.2-mm increase in cartilage thickness on MRI. In a prospective non-RCT open-label trial, 32 patients with severe grade III to IV OA were treated with lipoaspirate ASC. VAS, gadolinium MRI, and glycan content were assessed at baseline and 3, 6, and 12 months. There was a significant improvement in VAS sores at all time points compared with the baseline. MRI studies demonstrated an increase in glycan content.[94] In patients with severe OA, stem cells were collected from the Hoffa fat pad and injected into their knees.[95] The synovial fluid was then collected and analyzed with real-time polymerase chain reaction. After exposure to ASC, there was an increase in the expression of OPG, PTH1R, and MMP13.[95]

Koh and colleagues,[80] in 2015, published a small case trial of 30 patients who had ASC therapy from lipoaspirate. They followed up on these patients at 2 years assessing KOOS, VAS, and Lysholm scores as well as by performing a repeat diagnostic

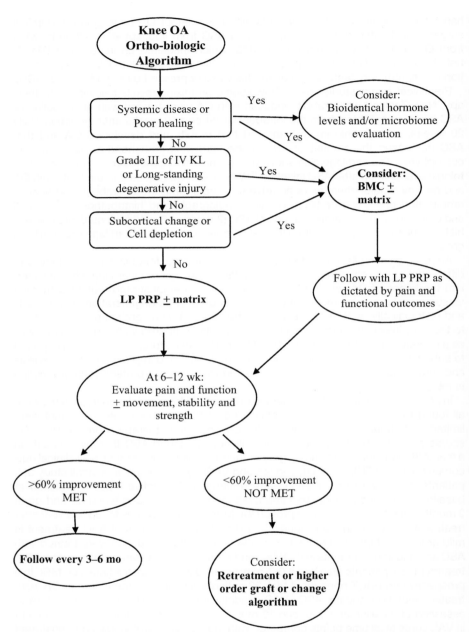

Fig. 1. Proposed algorithm for considering the use of ortho-biologics in OA as per Crane and colleagues. KL, kellgren lawrence. (*Data from* Crane DM, Oliver KS, Bayes MC. Orthobiologics and knee osteoarthritis: a recent literature review, treatment algorithm, and pathophysiology discussion. Phys Med Rehabil Clin N Am 2016;27(4):985–1002).

arthroscopic evaluation. Patients had a significant improvement in clinical outcomes. A total of 87.5% of patients had improved or maintained cartilage on arthroscopic evaluation, and most importantly none required a joint replacement over the study period.[67]

Although promising, these studies have been insufficient to draw conclusions about the efficacy of ASC therapy to adopt it into standard practices. These trials universally lack adequate controls and use a wide variety of approaches, injection regimes, and concentrations making it challenging to determine what would be the most efficacious and safest treatment going forward. In order to use evidence-based applications of ASC in OA, these gaps in knowledge must be studied and evaluated further.

DISCUSSION

In this article, the authors summarize what is known about the treatment of OA with regenerative medicine using 5 ortho-biologics: viscosupplementation, PRP, ACS, bone marrow aspirate concentrate and adipose-derived stromal cell therapy. All of these treatments have shown some promise in the literature; however, there are still substantial gaps in our knowledge. Guidelines for HA treatments have been less than enthusiastic; however, much of the data shows it to be safe and efficacious in patients with OA. Multiple meta-analyses of PRP treatments suggests that PRP is a promising therapy for symptom relief and improved functional outcomes in patients with OA for at least 12 months after treatment. Results of ACS therapy have been less conclusive than the use of PRP. Although there is some preliminary promise in the use of ACS in the treatment of OA, they have yet to reproduce the cytokine changes seen in vitro in humans. Cell therapies, including BMAC and ASC, are at the forefront of tissue engineering with lots of potential benefits in OA. These therapies are stem cell treatments, which are minimally manipulated allowing them to be used without further FDA regulations. With more studies, cell-based therapy may have the most promise when used appropriately in patients with OA.

Rapid advances in tissue engineering will make ortho-biologic therapies, particularly stem cell therapies, more feasible in changing the landscape of OA treatment. Crane and colleagues[96] have suggested that 15 factors will need to be considered going forward for both tissue engineering and treatment: tissue, neurohormonal status, vascular supply, growth factors, progenitor cells, matrix, cartilage, synovium, capsule, movement, stability, strength, tissue inflammation, hormones, and microbiome. Based on these criteria, they have proposed an algorithm for considering various ortho-biologic therapies (**Fig. 1**). Although this is an interesting algorithm, the lack of level 1 evidence to support these treatments makes it impossible at this stage to use this algorithm into daily practice.

In order to move forward with using these treatments, it is critical that we develop standardized study regimes that can be compared in large level 1 RCTs, meta-analyses, and systematic reviews.

SUMMARY

There have been large advancements in regenerative medicine in health care since the initial introduction of bone marrow therapies and PRP in the 1980s.[51,96] As regenerative medicine progresses, clinicians must make decisions on how best to optimize their use and when to use them based on the disease process and patients' treatment plan. This review demonstrates that the studies reviewed support that ortho-biologics are safe and seem to support their use in the treatment of OA for up to 2 years. These treatments are easy to obtain and relatively inexpensive. Ortho-biologics may yield superior results in the treatment of OA relative to more conventional approaches, because of their ability to target repair and regeneration of the underlying cartilage damage and dampen inflammation leading to this degradation.

Future work should be targeting the factors that are most beneficial and effective in treating OA, determining dosages and timing, in addition to administration methods. It is of the utmost importance that the medical community comes up with treatment algorithms and further trials studying long-term effectiveness.

REFERENCES

1. Foundation TA. 2018. Available at: https://www.arthritis.org/about-arthritis/types/osteoarthritis/what-is-osteoarthritis.php. Accessed February 20, 2018.
2. Woo J, Lau E, Lee P, et al. Impact of osteoarthritis on quality of life in a Hong Kong Chinese population. J Rheumatol 2004;31(12):2433–8.
3. Michael JW, Schluter-Brust KU, Eysel P. The epidemiology, etiology, diagnosis, and treatment of osteoarthritis of the knee. Dtsch Arztebl Int 2010;107(9):152–62.
4. Sakellariou VI, Poultsides LA, Ma Y, et al. Risk assessment for chronic pain and patient satisfaction after total knee arthroplasty. Orthopedics 2016;39(1):55–62.
5. AAOS. 2010. Available at: https://orthoinfo.aaos.org/en/treatment/helping-fractures-heal-orthobiologics.
6. Masuko K, Murata M, Yudoh K, et al. Anti-inflammatory effects of hyaluronan in arthritis therapy: not just for viscosity. Int J Gen Med 2009;2:77–81.
7. Moreland LW. Intra-articular hyaluronan (hyaluronic acid) and hylans for the treatment of osteoarthritis: mechanisms of action. Arthritis Res Ther 2003;5(2):54–67.
8. Stitik TP, Levy JA. Viscosupplementation (biosupplementation) for osteoarthritis. Am J Phys Med Rehabil 2006;85(11 Suppl):S32–50.
9. Altman R, Bedi A, Manjoo A, et al. Anti-inflammatory effects of intra-articular hyaluronic acid: a systematic review. Cartilage 2018. 1947603517749919. [Epub ahead of print].
10. Altman RD, Manjoo A, Fierlinger A, et al. The mechanism of action for hyaluronic acid treatment in the osteoarthritic knee: a systematic review. BMC Musculoskelet Disord 2015;16:321.
11. Rutjes AW, Juni P, da Costa BR, et al. Viscosupplementation for osteoarthritis of the knee: a systematic review and meta-analysis. Ann Intern Med 2012;157(3):180–91.
12. Miller LE, Block JE. US-approved intra-articular hyaluronic acid injections are safe and effective in patients with knee osteoarthritis: systematic review and meta-analysis of randomized, saline-controlled trials. Clin Med Insights Arthritis Musculoskelet Disord 2013;6:57–63.
13. Strand V, McIntyre LF, Beach WR, et al. Safety and efficacy of US-approved viscosupplements for knee osteoarthritis: a systematic review and meta-analysis of randomized, saline-controlled trials. J Pain Res 2015;8:217–28.
14. He WW, Kuang MJ, Zhao J, et al. Efficacy and safety of intraarticular hyaluronic acid and corticosteroid for knee osteoarthritis: a meta-analysis. Int J Surg 2017;39:95–103.
15. Euppayo T, Punyapornwithaya V, Chomdej S, et al. Effects of hyaluronic acid combined with anti-inflammatory drugs compared with hyaluronic acid alone, in clinical trials and experiments in osteoarthritis: a systematic review and meta-analysis. BMC Musculoskelet Disord 2017;18(1):387.

16. Bhandari M, Bannuru RR, Babins EM, et al. Intra-articular hyaluronic acid in the treatment of knee osteoarthritis: a Canadian evidence-based perspective. Ther Adv Musculoskelet Dis 2017;9(9):231–46.

17. Bannuru RR, Brodie CR, Sullivan MC, et al. Safety of repeated injections of sodium hyaluronate (SUPARTZ) for knee osteoarthritis: a systematic review and meta-analysis. Cartilage 2016;7(4):322–32.

18. Raman R, Henrotin Y, Chevalier X, et al. Decision algorithms for the retreatment with viscosupplementation in patients suffering from knee osteoarthritis: recommendations from the EUROpean VIScosupplementation COnsensus Group (EUROVISCO). Cartilage 2018;9(3):263–75.

19. Bhadra AK, Altman R, Dasa V, et al. Appropriate use criteria for hyaluronic acid in the treatment of knee osteoarthritis in the United States. Cartilage 2017;8(3): 234–54.

20. Sundman EA, Cole BJ, Karas V, et al. The anti-inflammatory and matrix restorative mechanisms of platelet-rich plasma in osteoarthritis. Am J Sports Med 2014; 42(1):35–41.

21. Anitua E, Sanchez M, Orive G. Potential of endogenous regenerative technology for in situ regenerative medicine. Adv Drug Deliv Rev 2010;62(7–8):741–52.

22. Arnoczky SP. Platelet-rich plasma augmentation of rotator cuff repair: letter. Am J Sports Med 2011;39(6):NP8–9 [author reply: NP9-11].

23. Mazzocca AD, McCarthy MB, Chowaniec DM, et al. Platelet-rich plasma differs according to preparation method and human variability. J Bone Joint Surg Am 2012;94(4):308–16.

24. Russell RP, Apostolakos J, Hirose T, et al. Variability of platelet-rich plasma preparations. Sports Med Arthrosc Rev 2013;21(4):186–90.

25. Werther K, Christensen IJ, Nielsen HJ. Determination of vascular endothelial growth factor (VEGF) in circulating blood: significance of VEGF in various leucocytes and platelets. Scand J Clin Lab Invest 2002;62(5):343–50.

26. Moojen DJ, Everts PA, Schure RM, et al. Antimicrobial activity of platelet-leukocyte gel against Staphylococcus aureus. J Orthop Res 2008;26(3):404–10.

27. Castillo TN, Pouliot MA, Kim HJ, et al. Comparison of growth factor and platelet concentration from commercial platelet-rich plasma separation systems. Am J Sports Med 2011;39(2):266–71.

28. DeLong JM, Russell RP, Mazzocca AD. Platelet-rich plasma: the PAW classification system. Arthroscopy 2012;28(7):998–1009.

29. Marx RE. Platelet-rich plasma (PRP): what is PRP and what is not PRP? Implant Dent 2001;10(4):225–8.

30. Akeda K, An HS, Okuma M, et al. Platelet-rich plasma stimulates porcine articular chondrocyte proliferation and matrix biosynthesis. Osteoarthritis Cartilage 2006; 14(12):1272–80.

31. Muraglia A, Ottonello C, Spano R, et al. Biological activity of a standardized freeze-dried platelet derivative to be used as cell culture medium supplement. Platelets 2014;25(3):211–20.

32. Wu CC, Chen WH, Zao B, et al. Regenerative potentials of platelet-rich plasma enhanced by collagen in retrieving pro-inflammatory cytokine-inhibited chondrogenesis. Biomaterials 2011;32(25):5847–54.

33. Kanwat H, Singh DM, Kumar CD, et al. The effect of intra-articular allogenic platelet rich plasma in Dunkin-Hartley guinea pig model of knee osteoarthritis. Muscles Ligaments Tendons J 2017;7(3):426–34.

34. Kwon DR, Park GY, Lee SU. The effects of intra-articular platelet-rich plasma injection according to the severity of collagenase-induced knee osteoarthritis in a rabbit model. Ann Rehabil Med 2012;36(4):458–65.

35. Ishida K, Kuroda R, Miwa M, et al. The regenerative effects of platelet-rich plasma on meniscal cells in vitro and its in vivo application with biodegradable gelatin hydrogel. Tissue Eng 2007;13(5):1103–12.

36. Anitua E, Sanchez M, Nurden AT, et al. Platelet-released growth factors enhance the secretion of hyaluronic acid and induce hepatocyte growth factor production by synovial fibroblasts from arthritic patients. Rheumatology (Oxford) 2007; 46(12):1769–72.

37. Cole BJ, Karas V, Hussey K, et al. Hyaluronic acid versus platelet-rich plasma: a prospective, double-blind randomized controlled trial comparing clinical outcomes and effects on intra-articular biology for the treatment of knee osteoarthritis. Am J Sports Med 2017;45(2):339–46.

38. Khatab S, van Buul GM, Kops N, et al. Intra-articular injections of platelet-rich plasma releasate reduce pain and synovial inflammation in a mouse model of osteoarthritis. Am J Sports Med 2018;46(4):977–86.

39. Sanchez M, Anitua E, Azofra J, et al. Intra-articular injection of an autologous preparation rich in growth factors for the treatment of knee OA: a retrospective cohort study. Clin Exp Rheumatol 2008;26(5):910–3.

40. Chang KV, Hung CY, Aliwarga F, et al. Comparative effectiveness of platelet-rich plasma injections for treating knee joint cartilage degenerative pathology: a systematic review and meta-analysis. Arch Phys Med Rehabil 2014;95(3):562–75.

41. Laudy AB, Bakker EW, Rekers M, et al. Efficacy of platelet-rich plasma injections in osteoarthritis of the knee: a systematic review and meta-analysis. Br J Sports Med 2015;49(10):657–72.

42. Riboh JC, Saltzman BM, Yanke AB, et al. Effect of leukocyte concentration on the efficacy of platelet-rich plasma in the treatment of knee osteoarthritis. Am J Sports Med 2016;44(3):792–800.

43. Meheux CJ, McCulloch PC, Lintner DM, et al. Efficacy of intra-articular platelet-rich plasma injections in knee osteoarthritis: a systematic review. Arthroscopy 2016;32(3):495–505.

44. Sadabad HN, Behzadifar M, Arasteh F, et al. Efficacy of platelet-rich plasma versus hyaluronic acid for treatment of knee osteoarthritis: a systematic review and meta-analysis. Electron Physician 2016;8(3):2115–22.

45. Dai WL, Zhou AG, Zhang H, et al. Efficacy of platelet-rich plasma in the treatment of knee osteoarthritis: a meta-analysis of randomized controlled trials. Arthroscopy 2017;33(3):659–70.e1.

46. Wassilew GI, Lehnigk U, Duda GN, et al. The expression of proinflammatory cytokines and matrix metalloproteinases in the synovial membranes of patients with osteoarthritis compared with traumatic knee disorders. Arthroscopy 2010;26(8): 1096–104.

47. Martel-Pelletier J, McCollum R, DiBattista J, et al. The interleukin-1 receptor in normal and osteoarthritic human articular chondrocytes. Identification as the type I receptor and analysis of binding kinetics and biologic function. Arthritis Rheum 1992;35(5):530–40.

48. Sadouk MB, Pelletier JP, Tardif G, et al. Human synovial fibroblasts coexpress IL-1 receptor type I and type II mRNA. The increased level of the IL-1 receptor in osteoarthritic cells is related to an increased level of the type I receptor. Lab Invest 1995;73(3):347–55.

49. Dinarello CA, Thompson RC. Blocking IL-1: interleukin 1 receptor antagonist in vivo and in vitro. Immunol Today 1991;12(11):404–10.
50. Dinarello CA. Interleukin-1. Rev Infect Dis 1984;6(1):51–95.
51. Meijer H, Reinecke J, Becker C, et al. The production of anti-inflammatory cytokines in whole blood by physico-chemical induction. Inflamm Res 2003;52(10): 404–7.
52. Baltzer AW, Moser C, Jansen SA, et al. Autologous conditioned serum (Orthokine) is an effective treatment for knee osteoarthritis. Osteoarthritis Cartilage 2009;17(2):152–60.
53. Auw Yang KG, Raijmakers NJ, van Arkel ER, et al. Autologous interleukin-1 receptor antagonist improves function and symptoms in osteoarthritis when compared to placebo in a prospective randomized controlled trial. Osteoarthritis Cartilage 2008;16(4):498–505.
54. Baselga Garcia-Escudero J, Miguel Hernandez Trillos P. Treatment of osteoarthritis of the knee with a combination of autologous conditioned serum and physiotherapy: a two-year observational study. PLoS One 2015;10(12):e0145551.
55. Rutgers M, Creemers LB, Auw Yang KG, et al. Osteoarthritis treatment using autologous conditioned serum after placebo. Acta Orthop 2015;86(1):114–8.
56. Barreto A, Braun TR. A new treatment for knee osteoarthritis: Clinical evidence for the efficacy of Arthrokinex autologous conditioned serum. J Orthop 2017;14(1): 4–9.
57. Smith PA. Intra-articular autologous conditioned plasma injections provide safe and efficacious treatment for knee osteoarthritis: an FDA-sanctioned, randomized, double-blind, placebo-controlled clinical trial. Am J Sports Med 2016; 44(4):884–91.
58. Zarringam D, Bekkers JEJ, Saris DBF. Long-term effect of injection treatment for osteoarthritis in the knee by orthokin autologous conditioned serum. Cartilage 2018;9(2):140–5.
59. Rutgers M, Saris DB, Dhert WJ, et al. Cytokine profile of autologous conditioned serum for treatment of osteoarthritis, in vitro effects on cartilage metabolism and intra-articular levels after injection. Arthritis Res Ther 2010;12(3):R114.
60. Jager M, Hernigou P, Zilkens C, et al. Cell therapy in bone healing disorders. Orthop Rev (Pavia) 2010;2(2):e20.
61. Muschler GF, Boehm C, Easley K. Aspiration to obtain osteoblast progenitor cells from human bone marrow: the influence of aspiration volume. J Bone Joint Surg Am 1997;79(11):1699–709.
62. Pierini M, Di Bella C, Dozza B, et al. The posterior iliac crest outperforms the anterior iliac crest when obtaining mesenchymal stem cells from bone marrow. J Bone Joint Surg Am 2013;95(12):1101–7.
63. Hernigou P, Homma Y, Flouzat Lachaniette CH, et al. Benefits of small volume and small syringe for bone marrow aspirations of mesenchymal stem cells. Int Orthop 2013;37(11):2279–87.
64. Caplan AI, Dennis JE. Mesenchymal stem cells as trophic mediators. J Cell Biochem 2006;98(5):1076–84.
65. Fortier LA, Potter HG, Rickey EJ, et al. Concentrated bone marrow aspirate improves full-thickness cartilage repair compared with microfracture in the equine model. J Bone Joint Surg Am 2010;92(10):1927–37.
66. Wakitani S, Imoto K, Yamamoto T, et al. Human autologous culture expanded bone marrow mesenchymal cell transplantation for repair of cartilage defects in osteoarthritic knees. Osteoarthritis Cartilage 2002;10(3):199–206.

67. Koh YG, Choi YJ, Kwon OR, et al. Second-look arthroscopic evaluation of cartilage lesions after mesenchymal stem cell implantation in osteoarthritic knees. Am J Sports Med 2014;42(7):1628–37.
68. Jo CH, Lee YG, Shin WH, et al. Intra-articular injection of mesenchymal stem cells for the treatment of osteoarthritis of the knee: a proof-of-concept clinical trial. Stem Cells 2014;32(5):1254–66.
69. Emadedin M, Aghdami N, Taghiyar L, et al. Intra-articular injection of autologous mesenchymal stem cells in six patients with knee osteoarthritis. Arch Iran Med 2012;15(7):422–8.
70. Orozco L, Munar A, Soler R, et al. Treatment of knee osteoarthritis with autologous mesenchymal stem cells: a pilot study. Transplantation 2013;95(12):1535–41.
71. Kim JD, Lee GW, Jung GH, et al. Clinical outcome of autologous bone marrow aspirates concentrate (BMAC) injection in degenerative arthritis of the knee. Eur J Orthop Surg Traumatol 2014;24(8):1505–11.
72. Shapiro SA, Kazmerchak SE, Heckman MG, et al. A prospective, single-blind, placebo-controlled trial of bone marrow aspirate concentrate for knee osteoarthritis. Am J Sports Med 2017;45(1):82–90.
73. Sampson S, Smith J, Vincent H, et al. Intra-articular bone marrow concentrate injection protocol: short-term efficacy in osteoarthritis. Regen Med 2016;11(6):511–20.
74. Centeno C, Pitts J, Al-Sayegh H, et al. Efficacy of autologous bone marrow concentrate for knee osteoarthritis with and without adipose graft. Biomed Res Int 2014;2014:370621.
75. Centeno CJ, Bashir J. Safety and regulatory issues regarding stem cell therapies: one clinic's perspective. PM R 2015;7(4 Suppl):S4–7.
76. Coughlin RP, Oldweiler A, Mickelson DT, et al. Adipose-derived stem cell transplant technique for degenerative joint disease. Arthrosc Tech 2017;6(5):e1761–6.
77. Garza JR, Santa Maria D, Palomera T, et al. Use of autologous adipose-derived stromal vascular fraction to treat osteoarthritis of the knee: a feasibility and safety study. J Regen Med 2015;4(1).
78. Maumus M, Manferdini C, Toupet K, et al. Adipose mesenchymal stem cells protect chondrocytes from degeneration associated with osteoarthritis. Stem Cell Res 2013;11(2):834–44.
79. Jin R, Shen M, Yu L, et al. Adipose-derived stem cells suppress inflammation induced by IL-1beta through down-regulation of P2X7R mediated by miR-373 in chondrocytes of osteoarthritis. Mol Cells 2017;40(3):222–9.
80. Koh YG, Choi YJ, Kwon SK, et al. Clinical results and second-look arthroscopic findings after treatment with adipose-derived stem cells for knee osteoarthritis. Knee Surg Sports Traumatol Arthrosc 2015;23(5):1308–16.
81. Bansal H, Comella K, Leon J, et al. Intra-articular injection in the knee of adipose derived stromal cells (stromal vascular fraction) and platelet rich plasma for osteoarthritis. J Transl Med 2017;15(1):141.
82. Manferdini C, Maumus M, Gabusi E, et al. Adipose-derived mesenchymal stem cells exert antiinflammatory effects on chondrocytes and synoviocytes from osteoarthritis patients through prostaglandin E2. Arthritis Rheum 2013;65(5):1271–81.
83. Toghraie FS, Chenari N, Gholipour MA, et al. Treatment of osteoarthritis with infrapatellar fat pad derived mesenchymal stem cells in Rabbit. Knee 2011;18(2):71–5.
84. Riester SM, Denbeigh JM, Lin Y, et al. Safety studies for use of adipose tissue-derived mesenchymal stromal/stem cells in a rabbit model for osteoarthritis to support a Phase I clinical trial. Stem Cells Transl Med 2017;6(3):910–22.

85. Parrilli A, Giavaresi G, Ferrari A, et al. Subchondral bone response to injected adipose-derived stromal cells for treating osteoarthritis using an experimental rabbit model. Biotech Histochem 2017;92(3):201–11.
86. Latief N, Raza FA, Bhatti FU, et al. Adipose stem cells differentiated chondrocytes regenerate damaged cartilage in rat model of osteoarthritis. Cell Biol Int 2016; 40(5):579–88.
87. Mei L, Shen B, Ling P, et al. Culture-expanded allogenic adipose tissue-derived stem cells attenuate cartilage degeneration in an experimental rat osteoarthritis model. PLoS One 2017;12(4):e0176107.
88. Mei L, Shen B, Xue J, et al. Adipose tissue-derived stem cells in combination with xanthan gum attenuate osteoarthritis progression in an experimental rat model. Biochem Biophys Res Commun 2017;494(1–2):285–91.
89. Tang Y, Pan ZY, Zou Y, et al. A comparative assessment of adipose-derived stem cells from subcutaneous and visceral fat as a potential cell source for knee osteoarthritis treatment. J Cell Mol Med 2017;21(9):2153–62.
90. Munoz-Criado I, Meseguer-Ripolles J, Mellado-Lopez M, et al. Human Suprapatellar fat pad-derived mesenchymal stem cells induce chondrogenesis and cartilage repair in a model of severe osteoarthritis. Stem Cells Int 2017;2017:4758930.
91. Pers YM, Rackwitz L, Ferreira R, et al. Adipose mesenchymal stromal cell-based therapy for severe osteoarthritis of the knee: a phase I dose-escalation trial. Stem Cells Transl Med 2016;5(7):847–56.
92. Russo A, Condello V, Madonna V, et al. Autologous and micro-fragmented adipose tissue for the treatment of diffuse degenerative knee osteoarthritis. J Exp Orthop 2017;4(1):33.
93. Fodor PB, Paulseth SG. Adipose derived stromal cell (ADSC) injections for pain management of osteoarthritis in the human knee joint. Aesthet Surg J 2016;36(2): 229–36.
94. Hudetz D, Boric I, Rod E, et al. The effect of intra-articular injection of autologous microfragmented fat tissue on proteoglycan synthesis in patients with knee osteoarthritis. Genes (Basel) 2017;8(10).
95. Bravo B, Arguello JM, Gortazar AR, et al. Modulation of gene expression in infrapatellar fat pad-derived mesenchymal stem cells in osteoarthritis. Cartilage 2018; 9(1):55–62.
96. Crane DM, Oliver KS, Bayes MC. Orthobiologics and knee osteoarthritis: a recent literature review, treatment algorithm, and pathophysiology discussion. Phys Med Rehabil Clin N Am 2016;27(4):985–1002.

Emerging Orthobiologic Techniques and the Future

Kevin Christensen, MD[a], Benjamin Cox, DO[b], Adam Anz, MD[c],*

KEYWORDS

• Orthobiologics • Future • Stem cells • PRP

KEY POINTS

- Ideal development of orthobiologics products should follow a developmental pyramid of evidence to prove safety and efficacy before widespread clinical application.
- Understanding regulatory classification and development is a key to translation of orthobiologics from animal study to clinical practice.
- There are emerging orthobiologics technologies that have followed the developmental pyramid; these will likely sustain the tests of time.

INTRODUCTION

Orthopedic sports medicine has advanced tremendously in the last 30 years, with most of the innovation surrounding the arthroscope and associated techniques. Advancement has been optimized when a pyramid of development has been pursued, and with Orthopedics, this has traditionally involved quantitative anatomy as the base, followed by biomechanical study, clinical application, revision with outcome data, and evidence-based clinical application at the pinnacle. The use of a developmental model has been termed translational biomechanics and illustrated as a pyramid. It has become clear that the next 30 years of advancements within sports medicine will involve the advancement of orthobiologics. A recent lesson is clear with one of the first orthobiologics, platelet-rich plasma (PRP). Clinical application without development leads to confusion among clinicians, industry, and patients about mechanism of action, safety, efficacy, and overall value. The future of orthobiologics lies in using a similar pyramid of development as translational biomechanics, with preclinical bench-top and animal studies at the base, followed by pilot clinical trials, controlled

Disclosure Statement: A. Anz receives research support, speaking reimbursement, and royalties from Arthrex. The Andrews Research and Education Foundation receives research support from Arthex and KLSMC Stem Cell.
[a] Andrews Institute, 1040 Gulf Breeze Parkway, Gulf Breeze, FL 32561, USA; [b] PLLC, 2890 Health Parkway, Mount Pleasant, MI 48858, USA; [c] Andrews Institute, Andrews Research and Education Foundation, 1040 Gulf Breeze Parkway, Gulf Breeze, FL 32561, USA
* Corresponding author.
E-mail address: anz.adam.w@gmail.com

Clin Sports Med 38 (2019) 143–161
https://doi.org/10.1016/j.csm.2018.08.007
0278-5919/19/© 2018 Elsevier Inc. All rights reserved.

comparative clinical trials, multicenter study, and clinical application at the pinnacle (**Fig. 1**).[1] Although daunting, expensive, and time consuming, developing this pyramid, sometimes called translational medicine, is the future of orthobiologics. Technologies that short-circuit the process will likely fade into history.

Clinical application of orthobiologics without development produces confusion and stagnates progress. Progress currently faces a delicate balance with providers and patients sprinting toward application of emerging technologies on one side and the marathon of technology development through translational medicine on the other side. Weighing the balance is the orthopedic community, the public, and government regulatory bodies. Scientists and clinicians must understand and embrace yet challenge the development pathway, to refine it, because the next steps of translation require patient care and clinician participation. A potential pitfall, industry may at times present biased interpretations of regulation and the developmental process to clinicians and patients, but ultimately patients as well as regulatory bodies expect physicians to understand the regulation of medical treatments that they offer. For this reason, this article reviews the principles of biologic product development and the regulation surrounding the development and discusses emerging technologies that are walking the path of development.

PRINCIPLES OF DEVELOPMENT FOR ORTHOBIOLOGICS

The foundational principles of development are mechanism of action, safety, and efficacy. Safety involves ensuring that in the course of administering a product in an appropriate fashion the product does not cause harm, injury, or loss by the recipient in a direct or indirect manner. For orthobiologics, safety often involves avoiding the possible introduction, spread, and/or transmission of infectious disease as well as ensuring that treatments do not cause undue adverse events. Adverse event concerns include the possibilities of immune reactions to biologic treatments, infections, the potential for neoplasms, and/or increasing the likelihood of a venous thromboembolic event. Efficacy generally involves the power of a treatment to produce a claimed effect. As new biologic treatments are emerging, the orthopedic community should consider that the due diligence of mechanism of action, safety, and efficacy should

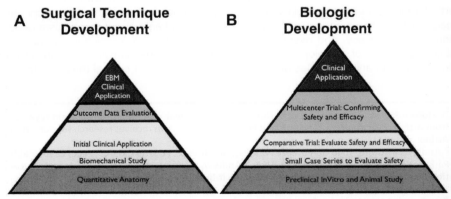

Fig. 1. (*A*) Translational biomechanics has been the developmental model of evidence-based orthopedic technique progress. (*B*) The future of orthobiologics will follow a similar developmental model. EBM, evidence based medicine. (*Courtesy of* Dr Adam Anz, Gulf Breeze, FL; with permission.)

precede marketing and/or making claims regarding biologic treatments. The Food and Drug Administration (FDA) was founded on the principle of ensuring that products are safe and effective before use as medical treatments. The FDA has been given the responsibility to protect the public from unproven treatments, and since 2008, the reach of the FDA has extended into both industry and the clinical practice of medicine regarding orthobiologics.

Monitoring and regulation of orthobiologics is a double-edged sword, important for patient safety and proof of worth on one side, but seemingly stifling to progress on the other. Loose regulation encourages clinical experimentation, but raises concerns for patient safety, and does not force products to prove their value before clinicians set prices, market, and use them for patient treatments. Although rigid regulation stifles progress, it ensures patient safety and forces technologies to prove themselves through a developmental process. The latter requires a significant investment of time and money, but produces clear indications and evidence for care.

FOOD AND DRUG ADMINISTRATION CLASSIFICATION OF ORTHOBIOLOGICS

Understanding the FDA's mechanisms is important for clinicians seeking to use orthobiologics and/or participate in the developmental process. To the FDA, most biological products are a subset of drugs,[2] and "biological" refers to those medical products that are derived from living material, as opposed to chemically synthesized.[2] The FDA does not consider everything that clinicians consider orthobiologics as biological products. The FDA applies the *Federal Food, Drug, and Cosmetic Act* for the monitoring and regulation of many orthobiologics especially those involving cells. The FDA derives its authority to regulate biologic products from the Public Health Service Act (PHSA), a federal law enacted in 1944 that outlines the federal government's duties to protect the health of the public. Section 351 of the PHSA (PHSA 351) addresses biological products defined as "virus, therapeutic serum, toxin, antitoxin, vaccine, blood, blood component or derivative, allergenic product, or analogous product, applicable to the prevention, treatment, or cure of a disease or condition of human beings."[2] PHSA 351 established the authority for the FDA's oversight in the development of these products. Section 361 of the PHSA (PHSA 361) granted the FDA the authority to prevent the spread of communicable diseases.

As biologics have emerged in medicine, the FDA has developed layered regulations, based on perceived risk to the United States Public, which set the mechanisms of control and oversight established in PHSA 351 and PHSA 361. These regulations are set forth in the Code of Federal Regulations. The Code of Federal Regulations is a document produced yearly that depicts the rules published in the Federal Register. These rules are established by the Executive departments and other agencies within the Federal Government. This document depicts the policies of the FDA and contains specific instructions to manufacturers, health care providers, and sponsors in the development/manufacture of products. Title 21 specifically focuses on the rules of the FDA. Part 1271 of Title 21 (21CFR 1271) is titled: Human Cells, Tissues, and Cellular and Tissue-based Products, or HCT/Ps for short, and addresses "articles containing or consisting of human cells or tissues that are intended for implantation transplantation, infusion, or transfer into a human recipient."

21CFR 1271 states that an HCT/P is regulated solely under 361 of the PHSA and must be manufactured to meet the requirements of 21 CFR 1271 alone if it meets 4 criteria: (1) the HCT/P is minimally manipulated; (2) the HCT/P is intended for homologous use only; (3) the manufacture of the HCT/P does not involve the combination of the cells or tissues with another article, except for water, crystalloids, or a sterilizing, preserving, or storage agent, provided that the addition of water, crystalloids, or the sterilizing, preserving, or storage agent does not raise new clinical safety concerns with respect to the HCT/P; (4) either the HCT/P does not have a systemic effect and is not dependent upon the metabolic activity of living cells for his primary function or if the HCT/P does have a systemic effect or is dependent upon the metabolic activity of living cells for its primary function, it is autologous or allogenic in a first-degree or second-degree blood relative (**Box 1**).[3] HCT/Ps that meet these 4 criteria are often termed "361 products." Whereas these HCT/Ps are not subject to premarket FDA review requirements, 1271 does set forth clear requirements within 6 domains: (1) registration and listing with the FDA, (2) donor screening and testing, (3) current good tissue practices, (4) labeling, (5) adverse-event reporting, and (6) inspection and enforcement. Certain exemptions for the requirements set in 1271 exist for some HCT/Ps, which are harvested, processed, and reimplanted in the same surgical procedure and are exempt from the requirements of CFR 1271; however, they are not exempt from overall regulation under PHSA 361 and/or 351. Guidance documents suggest that examples for exemption include veins harvested for coronary artery bypass grafting and cranial tissue harvested and stored for reimplantation at a later date.

HCT/Ps that do not meet criteria described in CFR 1271 are regulated as a drug under section 201(g) of the Federal Food, Drug, and Cosmetic Act, a device, and/or a biological product as outlined in PHSA 351 of the PHS Act. These products, often termed "351 products" are subject to premarket and postmarket development requirements and FDA approval before they can be marketed. In addition, their manufacture must comply with both current good tissue practices and current good manufacturing practices. Development requirements involve a series of steps often called the "351 pathway" and start with preclinical laboratory and animal testing to show that investigational use would be safe in humans. Before initiating clinical studies

---

Box 1
In order for an orthobiologic to be considered low risk by the Food and Drug Administration, it must meet 4 criteria

1. Minimal manipulation:
   The HCT/P is minimally manipulated

2. Homologous use:
   The HCT/P is intended for homologous use only, as reflected by the labeling, advertising, or other indications of the manufacturer's objective intent

3. None combination product:
   The manufacture of the HCT/P does not involve the combination of the cells or tissues with another article, except for water, crystalloids, or a sterilizing, preserving, or storage agent, provided that the addition of water, crystalloids, or the sterilizing, preserving, or storage agent does not raise new clinical safety concerns with respect to the HCT/P

4. None systemic effect or autologous:
   Either:
   i. The HCT/P does not have a systemic effect and is not dependent upon the metabolic activity of living cells for its primary function
   ii. The HCT/P has a systemic effect or is dependent upon the metabolic activity of living cells for its primary function, and
      a. Is for autologous use;
      b. Is for allogeneic use in a first-degree or second-degree blood relative; or
      c. Is for reproductive use.

Courtesy of Dr Adam Anz, Gulf Breeze, FL; with permission.

in humans, an investigational New Drug Application (IND) must be in place as described in 21 CFR 312. Subsequent clinical trials prove safety and efficacy in a phased fashion, most often first involving small pilot human study followed by large multicenter pivotal study. The FDA has illustrated recent flexibility in pathway design dependent on the product under development requiring only pilot and pivotal studies in some instances. Results demonstrating safety and efficacy for an indication are submitted to the FDA as part of a biologics license application (BLA). Approval of a BLA is required before marketing or administration of the product in clinical practice. Several milestones are recognized through the process, and the sponsor communicates with the FDA at multiple time points to guide the process.

Although orthopedists may consider it a surgical procedure, the FDA considers the process of taking tissue from an individual, processing the tissue, and replacing the tissue as the manufacture of a product.[4] It is important to highlight that, although PHSA 351 specifically states that blood or blood components are biologic products, the FDA has expressly stated that whole blood, blood components, and minimally manipulated bone marrow for homologous use are not considered HCT/Ps in guidance documents and has no precedent of regulating the application of these products by clinicians.[4] However, through untitled letters, warning letters, statements of the tissue reference group, and recently finalized guidance documents, the FDA has set precedent for autologous products produced from adipose tissue, allograft products derived from human placenta, allograft cell products, autologous cultured cell products, and autologous hematopoietic stem cells, suggesting that they regard these as 351 products. Although clinicians and industry may take liberty with interpretation in some instances citing a same surgical procedure exemption, the FDA has recently made clear statements removing ambiguity.[4,5]

In November 2017, the FDA released 2 guidance documents to aid clinicians and industry pertinent to orthobiologics. One document sought to clarify homologous use and minimal manipulation and used specific examples regarding adipose and placenta/amnion-derived products. This document clarified requirements of developmental process before clinical application.[4] The second document clarified the FDA's intent behind 21CFR1271.15(b), an exemption clause related to the setting of a surgical procedure. This document used the example of adipose tissue and stated that an establishment that harvests adipose tissue, processes the tissue by enzymatic or mechanical processes, and injects the product would not qualify for the exception.[5] Although the guidance documents are subject for interpretation, a subsequent publication in the *New England Journal of Medicine* authored by the director of the FDA's Center for Biologics Evaluation and Research and commissioner of the FDA clarifies the FDA's intent and interpretations. The FDA's goal is to facilitate innovation but ensure that emerging techniques prove they are safe and effective.[6]

EMERGING TECHNOLOGIES BUILDING A DEVELOPMENTAL PYRAMID

Although at times clinical application has outpaced development, there are many technologies that have leveraged the process to build a pyramid of developmental evidence. Review of a sample can help the clinician understand progress and gain a vision of the future of orthobiologics. Emerging techniques to treat osteoarthritis (OA), augment anterior cruciate ligament (ACL) repair/reconstruction, and improve cartilage repair have decades of developmental progress and represent the tip of the spear as well as technologies of the future.

Osteoarthritis

The first technology with a pyramid of development is point of care blood products, that is, PRP, for the indication of OA. At the top of this pyramid are recent systematic reviews and meta-analyses of comparative clinical trials that are clarifying a consensus that leukocyte-poor PRP is an effective intra-articular treatment for knee OA. The base of the pyramid began with animal and bench-top studies.

In bench-top studies, PRP has a clear mechanism of action to improve the catabolic and inflammatory environment of OA. Van Buul and colleagues[7] investigated the effects of PRP releasate upon cartilage cells that had been exposed to interleukin-1 (IL-1) beta, one of the most caustic inflammatory proteins within the osteoarthritic joint. They found that PRP releasate diminished multiple inflammatory effects of IL-1 on chondrocytes in culture, including reducing the activation of nuclear factor kappa B, a nuclear factor that upon activation translocates to the nucleus of cells and activates genes involved in apoptosis, inflammation, and other immune responses. Additional bench-top studies have shown that PRP stimulates proliferation of chondrocytes in culture,[8] decreases production of matrix metalloproteinases by synovial cells, and decreased inflammatory gene expression in an OA model.[9]

Preclinical animal studies have reflected bench-top progress. Saito and colleagues[10] investigated the effects of PRP on the progression of OA in a rabbit model. PRP in gelatin hydrogel microspheres was administered twice intra-articularly 4 weeks after ACL transection, a method to create a model of OA. At 10 weeks after the transection, cartilage samples illustrated superior histologic and morphologic scores in the PRP group, and the PRP group expressed significantly more proteoglycan messenger RNA. In a similar model, Yin and colleagues[11] evaluated the effects of a 3-PRP-injection regimen, comparing leukocyte-rich and leukocyte-poor PRP. Both the leukocyte-rich and the leukocyte-poor injections achieved better morphologic and histologic scores compared with a control, but the leukocyte-poor group had the best scores as well as reduced concentrations of inflammatory proteins. Similar study in mice involved an OA model created with intra-articular injection of a collagenase. A 3-injection series of PRP releasate reduced pain and synovial thickness when compared with a 3-injection series of saline.[12]

Clinical trials in humans have established safety and efficacy beginning with early small case series, followed by larger well-designed comparative cohort and randomized trials, and completing with systematic reviews of the literature. The orthopedic community is moving toward a consensus that intra-articular leukocyte-poor PRP is a safe and effective treatment for OA. A recent systematic review of the literature found 29 well-designed studies including 26 evaluating knee OA and 3 evaluating hip OA. The current status includes 9 prospective randomized controlled trials (RCTs), 8 knee and 1 hip, 4 prospective comparative studies, 14 case series, and 2 retrospective comparative studies. As a comparative group, hyaluronic acid (HA) was used as a control in 11 studies (7 RCTs, 2 prospective comparative studies, and 2 retrospective cohort). Only 2 RCTs, one for knee and one for hip, did not report significant superiority of PRP compared with the control group; in both of these studies, HA was used as a control. Nine out of 11 HA controlled studies showed significant better results in the PRP groups.[13]

One particular leukocyte-poor preparation deserves attention because it is progressing through clinical trials with the FDA, which will validate the technology to the entire orthopedic community, both national and international, as well as to payers. One company has developed a disposable that creates leukocyte-poor PRP, which they have branded as autologous conditioned plasma (ACP) and which is seeking an FDA approval. Clinical evaluation has 2 studies to highlight. Cerza and colleagues[14] compared the clinical response of HA to ACP in 2 groups of patients affected by knee OA. One hundred twenty patients were randomized to 2 groups: 60 patients received 4 weekly intra-articular injections of HA and 60 patients received 4 weekly injections of ACP. A significant effect was evident in the ACP group shortly after the final injection, and the effect improved up to 24 weeks (**Fig. 2**A).[14] Clinical outcomes were better than the results obtained with the HA based on Western Ontario and McMaster (WOMAC) score. ACP showed a significantly better clinical outcome than HA.[14] Development continued with a goal of FDA approval for knee OA beginning with an FDA-observed pilot study geared toward safety. One hundred fourteen patients were screened to yield 30 patients, randomized to 2 groups. A series of 3 weekly injections was studied, with saline as a control. WOMAC score served as the primary efficacy outcome measure, and patients were followed for 1 year. No adverse events were reported, and at conclusion, WOMAC scores for the ACP subjects had improved by 78% from baseline, whereas scores for the placebo group had improved by only 7% (**Fig. 2**B).[15]

Currently ACP is under multicenter evaluation for pivotal study. If the results of the pivotal study reflect the pilot data, an FDA approval can be expected. An FDA approval is the first step in obtaining CMS coverage and will provide leverage for the orthopedic community to seek reimbursement from private insurance companies. Because a developmental pyramid has been built, PRP is a technology that with continue to evolve, develop, and remain in the future, rather than a technology that will fade.

ANTERIOR CRUCIATE LIGAMENT REPAIR/RECONSTRUCTION

Another technology with developmental progress is the biologic augmentation of ACL repair and reconstruction. Martha Murray, MD, and her team at Boston Children's Hospital[16] have laid much of the instrumental preclinical groundwork, and progress to clinical

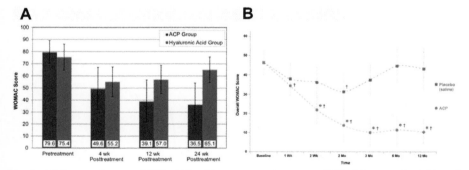

Fig. 2. (A) Results from an RCT in 120 subjects comparing mean WOMAC scores for ACP and HA groups. (B) Results of an FDA observed RCT in 30 subjects comparing a 3-weekly injection series of ACP to saline. Overall Western Ontario and McMaster Universities Osteoarthritis Index (WOMAC) scores versus time for the autologous conditioned plasma (ACP) and saline placebo treatment groups. * Significant difference from saline placebo (P \ .05); † Significant difference from baseline within each respective group (P \ .05). (From [A] Cerza F, Carnì S, Carcangiu A, et al. Comparison between hyaluronic acid and platelet-rich plasma, intra-articular infiltration in the treatment of gonarthrosis. Am J Sports Med 2012;40(12):2822–7, with permission; and [B] Smith PA. Intra-articular autologous conditioned plasma injections provide safe and efficacious treatment for knee osteoarthritis: an FDA-sanctioned, randomized, double-blind, placebo-controlled clinical trial. Am J Sports Med 2016;44(4):884–91, with permission.)

trials has been achieved. A central premise has emerged that a key to ACL healing and remodeling is providing an early, stable scaffold for the invasion of reparative cells. A key moment is a canine study evaluating a type-I collagen sponge loaded with a PRP hydrogel. A central defect was created in the ACL of a group of canines. Defect healing was evaluated with and without biologic enhancement. Repair tissue evaluated at 3 and 6 weeks showed better fill in the scaffold group at both 3 and 6 weeks. When tested biomechanically, the biologic scaffold group had 40% increased strength.[17]

Through preclinical research, development has continued clarifying the ideal initial repair construct, the best biologic addition, and appropriate metrics to evaluate healing. Regarding repair construct, Murray[18] found that bone to bone stabilization, with an internal splint, outperformed repair alone in a porcine model, improving the structural properties of healing tissue (**Fig. 3**). This concept has also been evaluated in a cadaver model of ACL reconstruction and found to significantly reduce elongation

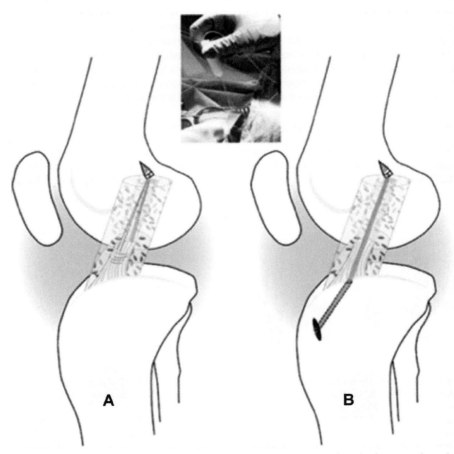

Fig. 3. A porcine animal model comparing ACL repair securing to the tibial stump alone (*A*) with repair including sutures through a tibial bone tunnel (*B*) found improved yield load and stiffness with the bone tunnel group but similar laxity in both groups. (*From* Murray MM, Magarian E, Zurakowski D, et al. Bone-to-bone fixation enhances functional healing of the porcine anterior cruciate ligament using a collagen-platelet composite. Arthroscopy 2010;26(9):S49–57. Figure 1; with permission.)

when cyclically loaded and produced a higher ultimate failure load without stress-shielding the graft.[19]

Different biologic enhancements have also been studied in preclinical development. In a minipig, bone-tendon-bone ACL reconstruction model, extracellular matrix (ECM) scaffolds were loaded with different PRP preparations. Although loading the scaffold with a PRP preparation similar to whole blood produced a biomechanically superior construct, loading a scaffold with increased platelet concentration PRP (3-fold and 5-fold) did not (**Fig. 4**).[20] Evaluating cultured cells in an ACL repair model, 3 methods of bioenhanced repair, an ECM matrix loaded with whole blood, an ECM matrix loaded with cells cultured from the fat pad, and an ECM matrix loaded with cells cultured from the buffy coat of whole blood were compared. After 15 weeks of healing, similar biomechanic and histologic properties were found between all groups, leading investigators to determine that whole blood is a sufficient biologic to augment repair and reconstruction.[21] Similar study has evaluated the biomechanic properties of tendon grafts loaded with bone marrow–derived cultured stem cells in a porcine model. Loading allograft tendons with cells and subjecting them to dynamic mechanical stimuli significantly enhanced matrix synthesis and ultimate tensile load after implantation.[22]

After refining bridge enhanced repair, Vavken and colleagues[23] compared repair to reconstruction in a porcine model. The repair group demonstrated no biomechanic difference and had less evidence of macroscopic cartilage damage when compared with reconstruction. Although biomechanic, morphologic, and histologic studies are sufficient outcome measures for preclinical animal studies, translation to human clinical trials requires noninvasive outcome measures. Biercevicz and colleagues[24,25]

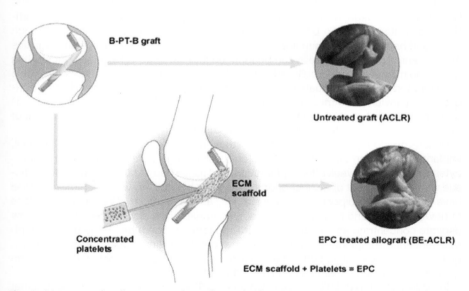

Fig. 4. Murray and colleagues evaluated standard ACL reconstruction to a bio-enhanced ACL reconstruction with differing concentrations of PRP. The scaffold is loaded with plasma containing a platelet concentration equal to blood performed superiorly when evaluated biomechanically. ACLR, anterior cruciate ligament reconstruction; BE-ACLR, bridge enhanced anterior cruciate ligament reconstruction; B-PT-B, bone patellar tendon bone. (*From* Fleming BC, Proffen BL, Vavken P, et al. Increased platelet concentration does not improve functional graft healing in bio-enhanced ACL reconstruction. Knee Surg Sports Traumatol Arthrosc 2015;23(4):1161–70; with permission.)

used 2 separate studies performed at Brown University to demonstrate that volume measurements and grayscale values from high-resolution T2 images were predictive of structural properties of ACL healing in a porcine model.

Murray began clinical study after an Investigational Device Exemption was obtained from the FDA.[26] A prospective cohort study compared bridge-enhanced ACL repair and standard autograft hamstring reconstruction. At 3-month follow up, neither group had any joint infections or signs of significant inflammation, and upon Lachman examination, the bridge-enhanced ACL repair had 8 International Knee Documentation Committee (IKDC) grade A examinations and 2 IKDC grade B examinations, whereas the ACL reconstruction group had 10 IKDC A examinations. MRIs from all patients demonstrated a continuous ACL or graft. Hamstring strength at 3 months was significantly better in the repair group. Longer follow-up will help clarify clinical performance. A similar, prospective randomized study is underway at the investigator's institution comparing standard ACL reconstruction to reconstruction augmented with a collagen matrix wrap seeded with bone marrow aspirate in both hamstring and patellar tendon ACL reconstructions (**Fig. 5**).[27]

Cartilage Repair

The largest developmental pyramid to date involves cartilage repair. Emerging techniques have been entrenched in development for decades, beginning with benchtop research, continuing with preclinical animal studies, and taking strides in the last decade through well-designed clinical trials. A clear pyramid of development has been built and guides emerging clinical application.

Although the earliest work on stem cells is attributed to Alexander Maximow at the University of Chicago in the 1920s,[28] foundational work applying stem cells to cartilage repair started on the bench top of Arnold Caplan in the late 1970s.[29] Through continued bench top and animal work all over the world, the mechanisms and logistics are becoming clear. Stem cells can be induced into cartilage cells, with work starting with bone marrow–derived cultured cells.[30] Cells from other tissue sources have also shown potential to differentiate to cartilage, including cells derived from adipose, periosteum, synovium, and muscle.[30–34] Because multiple cell sources have proven productive in bench-top study, the logistics around processing and application in light of regulatory/developmental requirements has guided further translation.

Bench-top work progressed to animal study in the early 1990s. In a rabbit model, implanted bone marrow–cultured MSCs on a collagen gel differentiated into chondrocytes by the second week after implantation, and tissue had organized into cartilage tissue with development of a subchondral bone plate by the 24th week.[35] Similar studies have followed with adipose,[36,37] synovium,[38,39] and periosteum.[40] With considerations of developmental and regulatory hurdles, researchers have also studied bone marrow aspirate concentrate as an adjunct to cartilage repair procedures. Bone marrow aspirate concentrate implanted at the time of a marrow stimulation procedure as a single implantation or series of injections after a marrow stimulation procedure have been shown to improve cartilage repair in an equine and caprine model.[41,42]

In addition to implantation of cells within a scaffold, another tested concept is that stem cells injected into a local environment, that is, a joint, have the potential to home (or localize) to an area of injury and participate in cartilage healing. Lee and colleagues[43] investigated this concept in a mini-pig. After the creation of a cartilage defect, one group received an intra-articular injection of stem cells cultured from bone marrow (BMSC) (average 7 million cells) suspended in HA followed by 2 additional weekly HA injections; another group received 3 weekly HA injections, and a third group received 3 weekly saline injections. Although both the HA and the BMSC groups were superior to saline, the

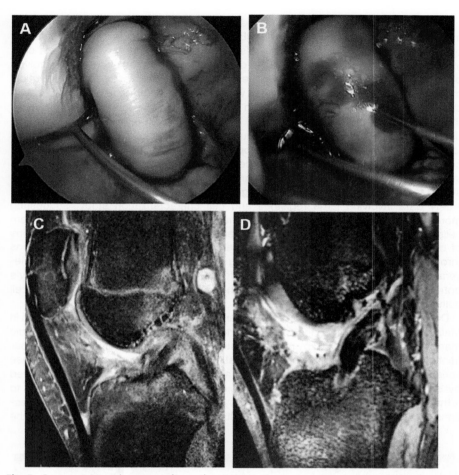

Fig. 5. Current RCT underway at the authors' institution comparing an ACL autograft wrapped with collagen matrix to a control group. Wrapped grafts are implanted (*A*) and then injected with bone marrow aspirate concentrate (*B*). MRI image of grafts in a control group (*C*) will be compared with intervention (*D*) at 3 months, 6 months, 12 months, and 24 months. (Original images from Steve Jordan, Adam Anz, James Andrews, unpublished data, 2018; and *Courtesy of* Dr Adam Anz, Gulf Breeze, FL; with permission.)

BMSC group stood out upon histologic and morphologic evaluation. The cells were also labeled with carboxyfluorescein, and upon histologic examination the labeled cells had homed to and integrated into the repair tissue. A similar study involving intra-articular injection of stem cells instead of direct open implantation has been performed with the same conclusions drawn in a meniscus injury model involving cultured synovial derived stem cells[44] and a large-animal model involving BMSC.[45]

Standing on a broad base of preclinical evidence, human studies have emerged and continue to emerge in 3 phases: case report/series design, comparative treatment study, and randomized controlled study. Recent systematic review found 60 clinical studies, including 9 case reports, 31 case series, 13 comparative trials, and 7 randomized controlled studies.[13] Stem cell treatments for cartilage repair are emerging as a safe and effective treatment, yet further well-designed comparative study is needed.

One stem cell technology that has been developing through FDA trials involves mobilized peripheral blood stem cells (PBSC). This technology follows the footsteps of the hematology oncology profession's development of the harvest of stem cells for bone marrow transplant. Although originally bone marrow transplant involved bone marrow aspiration harvest, the profession developed harvest via pharmaceutical mobilization followed by venous harvest with apheresis. Pharmaceutical mobilization stimulates an upregulation of production of cells in the bone marrow and release of these cells to the peripheral circulation. Apheresis harvest involves a machine that uses centrifugation, optics, and continuous venous access for a period of 1 to 4 hours to collect PBSC. For example, with orthopedic indications in mind, a 140-mL harvest contains on average 140 million CD34[+] cells, a quality control marker used to monitor stem cell numbers for bone marrow transplant. The harvest can be aliquoted and stored for serial/multiple injections[46] (**Fig. 6**).[47] These cell sources have established safety data involving large registries and cell characterization study, suggesting more immaturity than BMSC and functional properties similar to embryonal stem cells.[48,49] One striking advantage of this cell source is the ability to harvest millions of cells at one time point, which can be aliquoted and stored for serial injections throughout the maturation phase of cartilage healing. In addition, this technology leverages established techniques developed for bone marrow transplant and the body's potential to create stem cells to produce hundreds of millions of cells, without cell culture.

Developmental work applying PBSC to cartilage repair has emerged from a group in Malaysia. Lee and colleagues[43] first reported a case series involving arthroscopic marrow stimulation followed by multiple postoperative intra-articular injections in 5 patients, with safety data and histology suggesting good cartilage repair tissue. The case series was followed by an RCT comparing arthroscopic marrow stimulation followed by 8 postoperative PBSC intra-articular injections over the course of 6 months to arthroscopic marrow stimulation followed by 8 postoperative HA intra-articular injections. At 2 years, histology and MRI results favored the treatment group, and the

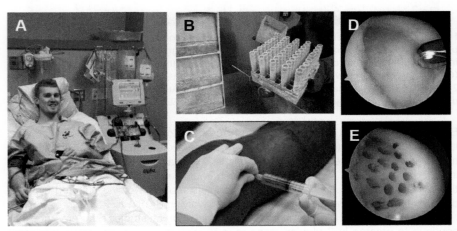

Fig. 6. After aphaeresis harvest (*A*), aliquoting and cryopreservation of mobilized PBSCs (*B*) allow for harvest at one time point and multiple injections (*C*) after arthroscopic subchondral drilling of large cartilage defects (*D, E*). (*From* Saw KY, Anz A, Jee CSY, et al. High tibial osteotomy in combination with chondrogenesis after stem cell therapy: a histologic report of 8 cases. Arthroscopy 2015;31(10):1909–20; with permission.)

clinical outcomes scores did not reveal superiority. On average, each stem cell injection in the intervention group contained 8 million stem cells.[50] This group recently published a case series combining the cartilage procedure with high tibial osteotomy.[47] Repair cartilage in this combination produced the best histology to date, and when graded with the ICRS scoring system, the cartilage repair score approached 95% of a normal articular cartilage control (**Fig. 7**).[47] Removing the deforming force responsible for cartilage wear is a key lesson learned. Similar encouraging results have been seen in 2 additional case series involving PBSC and one comparative study of open implantation of PBSC to BMC.[51–53] A multicenter, randomized study is underway in the United States with an IND Application reviewed and approved by the FDA.

A similar technology involving adipose-derived cells for cartilage repair is emerging from a group out of South Korea. Studies initiated with harvesting adipose from the infrapatellar fat pad and settled with liposuction harvest from the buttock region.[54] The methodology for the group involves processing the tissue with centrifugation and a collagenase to digest tissue. It reliably produces 4 million ADSCs from 120 mL of lipoaspirate. The group has investigated one administration time point via intra-articular injection, arthroscopic implantation without a scaffold with PRP, and arthroscopic implantation with a fibrin scaffold. Arthroscopic implantation with a fibrin scaffold has proven safe and the most effective method for administration of this cell product. They have shown that it can improve the clinical results of simple arthroscopic debridement, marrow stimulation, and osteotomy. Comparative study to additional cartilage repair technologies is lacking. This group has reported significant clinical and morphologic improvement when evaluated with MRI; yet histologic results have shown room for further development. These investigators have determined that older age, higher body mass index, and a larger defect size were negative predictors in all studies.[55–62]

THE FUTURE OF ORTHOBIOLOGICS: REGULATORY EVOLUTION

Historically, the FDA has been the global leader of medical regulation. Industrialized nations including but not limited to the European Union, Canada, and Australia have

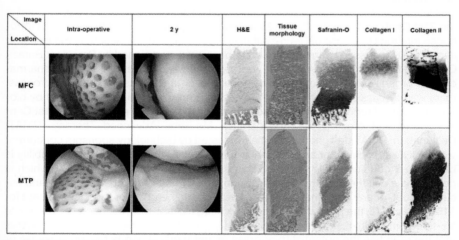

Fig. 7. Findings of second-look arthroscopy and histologic assessment of medial femoral condyle (MFC) and medial tibial plateau (MTP) at 2 years in a 49-year-old male patient. (*From* Saw KY, Anz A, Jee CSY, et al. High tibial osteotomy in combination with chondrogenesis after stem cell therapy: a histologic report of 8 cases. Arthroscopy 2015;31(10):1909–20; with permission.)

traditionally followed their guidance. The strict methods applied by the FDA have created a vacuum as technologies around stem cells have emerged. Although a few clinicians have taken advantage of underdeveloped countries to offer products not available in the United States, including cultured cells and cells from placenta tissue, this is not the norm outside of the United States in developed countries nor in the global stem cell community. The developed world sees the need for regulation in this space to protect vulnerable patients from unproven technologies and regulatory evolution is the key to translating these technologies to patient care.[63]

Regulatory evolution is the future and has begun. In 2014, Japan differentiated stem cell therapies from other pharmaceuticals by referring to these cell treatments as "regenerative medicine products." A new approval system was created and allowed early observed commercialization with reimbursement following a much less demanding safety and efficacy review. With this less demanding system, developing therapies can financially support some of the final most expensive clinical trials through early observed commercialization. With this change in regulation, Japan has positioned them to be leaders in this expanding field of research and development.

In March 2016, an attempt to evolve the US approval system was made. The Reliable and Effective Growth for Regenerative Health Options that Improve Wellness (REGROW) Act was proposed both to the United States Senate and to the House of Representatives and proposed a change in regulation that mirrored Japan's regulatory change. The REGROW Act proposed an addition to the PHSA, section 351B, to specifically address emerging technologies. Section 351B would have allowed for a conditional approval after certain developmental milestones. Specifically, following appropriate animal studies, completion of phase 1 testing, and early results of phase 2 testing, a conditional approval would have been granted to allow the sponsor of the therapy to treat patients and market the therapy during a 5-year trial period. At the end of the 5-year trial, the sponsor would apply for approval of the product as a biologic product. The goal of the addition would be to lower the initial financial hurdle of premarket development steps while still requiring the technologies to prove safety and efficacy.[64]

In late 2016, the discussion and direction of the REGROW Act became enveloped in the 21st Century Cures Act.[64] The 21st Century Cures Act is a bill that was first introduced into the US House of Representatives in January 2015, passed by the House in January 2016, passed by the Senate in October 2016, and signed by President Barack Obama in December 2016. This Act was supported and influenced by large pharmaceutical organizations and opposed by consumer organizations. Through the process, there was discussion about the creation of 351B; however, this was opposed by biopharmaceutical representatives. Instead of creating the 351B pathway, the 21st Century Cures Act created the Regenerative Medicine Advanced Therapy (RMAT) Designation. RMAT designation can be requested by technology sponsors concurrent with an IND application or as an amendment to an IND application. RMAT eligibility is based on 3 conditions: (1) the product is a regenerative medicine therapy, which is defined as a cell therapy, therapeutic tissue engineering product, human cell and tissue product, or any combination product using such therapies or products, except for 316 products; (2) the product is intended to treat, modify, reverse, or cure a serious or life-threatening disease or condition; and (3) preliminary clinical evidence indicates that the drug has the potential to address unmet medical needs for such disease or condition. The FDA upon determination that the technology meets the requirements allows for the treatment to enter one of the FDA's 4 expedited programs for serious conditions.[65] In addition, under certain circumstances, the Act allows for companies to use observational studies, insurance claim data, patient input data, and level V evidence as opposed to traditional drug trial design.[66] Time will determine whether the RMAT designation is sufficient evolution to improve the translation potential for orthobiologics; however, it is likely that further refinement of the regulation pathway and future legislation or executive direction will be necessary. It is important for orthopedic clinicians and leaders to understand the current regulatory environment and progress in order to participate in the refinement.

SUMMARY

Although the past is marked by murky regulation and the market of unproven treatments, the future of biologics within orthopedics is brighter and clearer with development. Through the developmental pyramid, PRP has proven that it will continue to be a part of the treatment of OA and appears close to an FDA approval for this indication. Similar progress in the biology of ACL surgery is being made, with studies showing the value of an internal splint, scaffolds, and biologic enhancement. Emerging cartilage repair technologies have the largest pyramid of development and are progressing through the FDA approval pathway. In summation, a key has been and will continue to be the developmental process, and reviewing recent paths provides an excellent roadmap for similar emerging therapies.[26] The future will require regulatory involvement and the developmental process both keys for widespread acceptance, payer reimbursement, and accepted clinical application. In light of this fact, regulatory bodies and payers must evolve to expedite the process.

Clinical practice should not outpace evidence regarding safety and efficacy. It is important to remember that patients do represent a vulnerable population, and influencing forces in the orthobiologic space include hope, hype, logistics, and truth. Technologies without transparent development will fade and be replaced by those that performed the necessary steps of development. The orthopedic community must remain grounded in evidence and truth, instead of seeking to profit on the vulnerability of patients by marketing unproven treatments. There is a thick gray area when applying orthobiologics. To navigate, providers should review FDA guidance documents, evaluate the evidence behind technologies, and last, consider the physical risk to the patient and the judicial/regulator risk to the provider. As always, the endless pursuit of well-designed clinical trials and animal studies remains the future for our understanding, and there always remains more to learn. In this space, it is key to stay green and remember: "If you are green, you are still growing. If you are ripe, you are next to rotten."

REFERENCES

1. Anz A. Figure 1: Translational pyramid.
2. Research C for DE and. Therapeutic Biologic Applications (BLA) - Frequently Asked Questions About Therapeutic Biological Products. Available at: https://www.fda.gov/drugs/developmentapprovalprocess/howdrugsaredevelopedand approved/approvalapplications/therapeuticbiologicapplications/ucm113522.htm. Accessed April 8, 2018.
3. Anz A. Figure 2: 4 criteria for biologic regulation under PHSA 361 and 21 CFR 1271 alone.
4. Regulatory Considerations for Human Cells, Tissues, and Cellular and Tissue-Based Products: Minimal Manipulation and Homologous Use. Available at: https://www.fda.gov/downloads/BiologicsBloodVaccines/GuidanceCompliance RegulatoryInformation/Guidances/CellularandGeneTherapy/UCM585403.pdf. Accessed April 8, 2018.

5. Same Surgical Procedure Exception under 21 CFR 1271.15(b): Questions and Answers Regarding the Scope of the Exception. Available at: https://www.fda.gov/downloads/BiologicsBloodVaccines/GuidanceComplianceRegulatoryInformation/Guidances/Tissue/UCM419926.pdf. Accessed April 8, 2018.
6. Marks P, Gottlieb S. Balancing safety and innovation for cell-based regenerative medicine. N Engl J Med 2018;378(10):954–9.
7. van Buul GM, Koevoet WLM, Kops N, et al. Platelet-rich plasma releasate inhibits inflammatory processes in osteoarthritic chondrocytes. Am J Sports Med 2011;39(11):2362–70.
8. Cavallo C, Filardo G, Mariani E, et al. Comparison of Platelet-Rich plasma formulations for cartilage healing: an in vitro study. J Bone Joint Surg Am 2014;96(5):423–9.
9. Osterman C, McCarthy MBR, Cote MP, et al. Platelet-Rich plasma increases anti-inflammatory markers in a human coculture model for osteoarthritis. Am J Sports Med 2015;43(6):1474–84.
10. Saito M, Takahashi KA, Arai E, et al. Intra-articular administration of platelet-rich plasma with biodegradable gelatin hydrogel microspheres prevents osteoarthritis progression in the rabbit knee. Clin Exp Rheumatol 2009;27(2):201.
11. Yin W-J, Xu H-T, Sheng J-G, et al. Advantages of pure Platelet-Rich plasma compared with leukocyte- and platelet-rich plasma in treating rabbit knee osteoarthritis. Med Sci Monit 2016;22:1280–90.
12. Khatab S, van Buul GM, Kops N, et al. Intra-articular Injections of platelet-rich plasma releasate reduce pain and synovial inflammation in a mouse model of osteoarthritis. Am J Sports Med 2018;46(4):977–86.
13. Filardo G, Perdisa F, Roffi A, et al. Stem cells in articular cartilage regeneration. J Orthop Surg Res 2016;11:42.
14. Cerza F, Carnì S, Carcangiu A, et al. Comparison between hyaluronic acid and platelet-rich plasma, intra-articular infiltration in the treatment of gonarthrosis. Am J Sports Med 2012;40(12):2822–7.
15. Smith PA. Intra-articular autologous conditioned plasma injections provide safe and efficacious treatment for knee osteoarthritis: an FDA-sanctioned, randomized, double-blind, placebo-controlled clinical trial. Am J Sports Med 2016;44(4):884–91.
16. Murray MM. Current status and potential of primary ACL repair. Clin Sports Med 2009;28(1):51–61.
17. Murray MM, Spindler KP, Devin C, et al. Use of a collagen-platelet rich plasma scaffold to stimulate healing of a central defect in the canine ACL. J Orthop Res 2006;24(4):820–30.
18. Murray MM, Magarian E, Zurakowski D, et al. Bone-to-bone fixation enhances functional healing of the porcine anterior cruciate ligament using a collagen-platelet composite. Arthroscopy 2010;26(9):S49–57.
19. Bachmaier S, Smith PA, Bley J, et al. Independent suture tape reinforcement of small and standard diameter grafts for anterior cruciate ligament reconstruction: a biomechanical full construct model. Arthrosc J Arthrosc Relat Surg 2018;34(2):490–9.
20. Fleming BC, Proffen BL, Vavken P, et al. Increased platelet concentration does not improve functional graft healing in bio-enhanced ACL reconstruction. Knee Surg Sports Traumatol Arthrosc 2015;23(4):1161–70.
21. Proffen BL, Vavken P, Haslauer CM, et al. Addition of autologous mesenchymal stem cells to whole blood for bioenhanced ACI repair has no benefit in the porcine model. Am J Sports Med 2015;43(2):320–30.

22. Lee KI, Lee JS, Kang KT, et al. In vitro and in vivo performance of tissue-engineered tendons for anterior cruciate ligament reconstruction. Am J Sports Med 2018. https://doi.org/10.1177/0363546518759729. 036354651875972.
23. Vavken P, Fleming BC, Mastrangelo AN, et al. Biomechanical outcomes after bio-enhanced anterior cruciate ligament repair and anterior cruciate ligament reconstruction are equal in a porcine model. Arthrosc J Arthrosc Relat Surg 2012;28(5): 672–80.
24. Biercevicz AM, Miranda DL, Machan JT, et al. In situ, noninvasive, T2*-weighted MRI-derived parameters predict ex vivo structural properties of an anterior cruciate ligament reconstruction or bioenhanced primary repair in a porcine model. Am J Sports Med 2013;41(3):560–6.
25. Biercevicz AM, Proffen BL, Murray MM, et al. T_2* relaxometry and volume predict semi-quantitative histological scoring of an ACL bridge-enhanced primary repair in a porcine model: MRI ACL HISTOLOGY. J Orthop Res 2015;33(8): 1180–7.
26. Proffen BL, Perrone GS, Roberts G, et al. Bridge-enhanced ACL repair: a review of the science and the pathway through FDA investigational device approval. Ann Biomed Eng 2015;43(3):805–18.
27. Anz A. Figure 6.
28. Maximow AA. Development of non-granular leucocytes (lymphocytes and monocytes) into polyblasts (macrophages) and fibroblasts in vitro. Proc Soc Exp Biol Med 1927;24(6):570–2.
29. Caplan AI. Review: mesenchymal stem cells: cell-based reconstructive therapy in orthopedics. Tissue Eng 2005;11(7–8):1198–211.
30. Johnstone B, Hering TM, Caplan AI, et al. In vitro chondrogenesis of bone marrow-derived mesenchymal progenitor cells. Exp Cell Res 1998;238(1): 265–72.
31. Dragoo JL, Samimi B, Zhu M, et al. Tissue-engineered cartilage and bone using stem cells from human infrapatellar fat pads. J Bone Joint Surg Br 2003;85(5): 740–7.
32. De Bari C, Dell'Accio F, Tylzanowski P, et al. Multipotent mesenchymal stem cells from adult human synovial membrane. Arthritis Rheum 2001;44(8):1928–42.
33. Sakaguchi Y, Sekiya I, Yagishita K, et al. Comparison of human stem cells derived from various mesenchymal tissues: superiority of synovium as a cell source. Arthritis Rheum 2005;52(8):2521–9.
34. Jiang Y, Cai Y, Zhang W, et al. Human cartilage-derived progenitor cells from committed chondrocytes for efficient cartilage repair and regeneration. Stem Cells Transl Med 2016;5(6):733–44.
35. Wakitani S, Goto T, Pineda SJ, et al. Mesenchymal cell-based repair of large, full-thickness defects of articular cartilage. J Bone Joint Surg Am 1994;76(4):579–92.
36. Dragoo JL, Carlson G, McCormick F, et al. Healing full-thickness cartilage defects using adipose-derived stem cells. Tissue Eng 2007;13(7):1615–21.
37. Masuoka K, Asazuma T, Hattori H, et al. Tissue engineering of articular cartilage with autologous cultured adipose tissue-derived stromal cells using atelocollagen honeycomb-shaped scaffold with a membrane sealing in rabbits. J Biomed Mater Res B Appl Biomater 2006;79(1):25–34.
38. Nakamura T, Sekiya I, Muneta T, et al. Arthroscopic, histological and MRI analyses of cartilage repair after a minimally invasive method of transplantation of allogeneic synovial mesenchymal stromal cells into cartilage defects in pigs. Cytotherapy 2012;14(3):327–38.

39. Koga H, Muneta T, Ju Y-J, et al. Synovial stem cells are regionally specified according to local microenvironments after implantation for cartilage regeneration. Stem Cells 2007;25(3):689–96.

40. Martin-Hernandez C, Cebamanos-Celma J, Molina-Ros A, et al. Regenerated cartilage produced by autogenous periosteal grafts: a histologic and mechanical study in rabbits under the influence of continuous passive motion. Arthroscopy 2010;26(1):76–83.

41. Fortier LA, Potter HG, Rickey EJ, et al. Concentrated bone marrow aspirate improves full-thickness cartilage repair compared with microfracture in the equine model. J Bone Joint Surg Am 2010;92(10):1927–37.

42. Saw K-Y, Hussin P, Loke S-C, et al. Articular cartilage regeneration with autologous marrow aspirate and hyaluronic Acid: an experimental study in a goat model. Arthroscopy 2009;25(12):1391–400.

43. Lee KBL, Hui JHP, Song IC, et al. Injectable mesenchymal stem cell therapy for large cartilage defects–a porcine model. Stem Cells 2007;25(11):2964–71.

44. Horie M, Sekiya I, Muneta T, et al. Intra-articular Injected synovial stem cells differentiate into meniscal cells directly and promote meniscal regeneration without mobilization to distant organs in rat massive meniscal defect. Stem Cells 2009;27(4):878–87.

45. McIlwraith CW, Frisbie DD, Rodkey WG, et al. Evaluation of intra-articular mesenchymal stem cells to augment healing of microfractured chondral defects. Arthroscopy 2011;27(11):1552–61.

46. Saw K-Y, Anz A, Merican S, et al. Articular cartilage regeneration with autologous peripheral blood progenitor cells and hyaluronic acid after arthroscopic subchondral drilling: a report of 5 cases with histology. Arthrosc J Arthrosc Relat Surg 2011;27(4):493–506.

47. Saw K-Y, Anz A, Jee CS-Y, et al. High tibial osteotomy in combination with chondrogenesis after stem cell therapy: a histologic report of 8 cases. Arthroscopy 2015;31(10):1909–20.

48. Cesselli D, Beltrami AP, Rigo S, et al. Multipotent progenitor cells are present in human peripheral blood. Circ Res 2009;104(10):1225–34.

49. Holig K, Kramer M, Kroschinsky F, et al. Safety and efficacy of hematopoietic stem cell collection from mobilized peripheral blood in unrelated volunteers: 12 years of single-center experience in 3928 donors. Blood 2009;114(18):3757–63.

50. Saw K-Y, Anz A, Siew-Yoke Jee C, et al. Articular cartilage regeneration with autologous peripheral blood stem cells versus hyaluronic acid: a randomized controlled trial. Arthrosc J Arthrosc Relat Surg 2013;29(4):684–94.

51. Turajane T, Chaweewannakorn U, Larbpaiboonpong V, et al. Combination of intra-articular autologous activated peripheral blood stem cells with growth factor addition/preservation and hyaluronic acid in conjunction with arthroscopic microdrilling mesenchymal cell stimulation Improves quality of life and regenerates articular cartilage in early osteoarthritic knee disease. J Med Assoc Thai 2013;96(5):580–8.

52. Fu W-L, Ao Y-F, Ke X-Y, et al. Repair of large full-thickness cartilage defect by activating endogenous peripheral blood stem cells and autologous periosteum flap transplantation combined with patellofemoral realignment. Knee 2014;21(2):609–12.

53. Skowroński J, Skowroński R, Rutka M. Cartilage lesions of the knee treated with blood mesenchymal stem cells - results. Ortop Traumatol Rehabil 2012;14(6):569–77.

54. Koh Y-G, Choi Y-J. Infrapatellar fat pad-derived mesenchymal stem cell therapy for knee osteoarthritis. Knee 2012;19(6):902–7.
55. Koh Y-G, Choi Y-J, Kwon S-K, et al. Clinical results and second-look arthroscopic findings after treatment with adipose-derived stem cells for knee osteoarthritis. Knee Surg Sports Traumatol Arthrosc 2015;23(5):1308–16.
56. Kim YS, Park EH, Kim YC, et al. Clinical outcomes of mesenchymal stem cell injection with arthroscopic treatment in older patients with osteochondral lesions of the talus. Am J Sports Med 2013;41(5):1090–9.
57. Koh Y-G, Kwon O-R, Kim Y-S, et al. Adipose-derived mesenchymal stem cells with microfracture versus microfracture alone: 2-year follow-up of a prospective randomized trial. Arthrosc J Arthrosc Relat Surg 2016;32(1):97–109.
58. Koh YG, Choi YJ, Kwon OR, et al. Second-look arthroscopic evaluation of cartilage lesions after mesenchymal stem cell implantation in osteoarthritic knees. Am J Sports Med 2014;42(7):1628–37.
59. Kim YS, Choi YJ, Suh DS, et al. Mesenchymal stem cell implantation in osteoarthritic knees: is fibrin glue effective as a scaffold? Am J Sports Med 2015;43(1):176–85.
60. Kim YS, Lee HJ, Choi YJ, et al. Does an injection of a stromal vascular fraction containing adipose-derived mesenchymal stem cells influence the outcomes of marrow stimulation in osteochondral lesions of the talus?: a clinical and magnetic resonance imaging study. Am J Sports Med 2014;42(10):2424–34.
61. Kim YS, Choi YJ, Koh YG. Mesenchymal stem cell implantation in knee osteoarthritis: an assessment of the factors influencing clinical outcomes. Am J Sports Med 2015;43(9):2293–301.
62. Kim YS, Choi YJ, Lee SW, et al. Assessment of clinical and MRI outcomes after mesenchymal stem cell implantation in patients with knee osteoarthritis: a prospective study. Osteoarthritis Cartilage 2016;24(2):237–45.
63. Policy & Advocacy. Available at: http://www.isscr.org/membership/policy. Accessed April 13, 2018.
64. Kirk M. S.2689 - 268114th Congress (2015-2016): REGROW Act. 2016. Available at: https://www.congress.gov/bill/114th-congress/senate-bill/2689. Accessed April 13, 2018.
65. Expedited Programs for Serious Conditions – Drugs and Biologics. Available at: https://www.fda.gov/downloads/drugs/guidancecomplianceregulatoryinformation/guidances/ucm358301.pdf. Accessed April 13, 2018.
66. Inside the 21st Century Cures Act | Cancer Today. Available at: https://www.cancertodaymag.org/pages/Spring2017/Inside-the-21st-Century-Cures-Act.aspx. Accessed April 13, 2018.

Incorporating Ortho-Biologics into Your Clinical Practice

Colin P. Murphy, BA[a,1], Anthony Sanchez, BS[a,b,2],
Liam A. Peebles, BA[a,3], Matthew T. Provencher, MD[a,c],*

KEYWORDS

- Ortho-biologics • Platelet-rich plasma (PRP) • Demineralized bone matrix (DBM)
- Mesenchymal stem cells (MSCs) • Allograft bone products
- Synthetic bone graft substitutes • Bone marrow aspirate concentrate (BMAC)

KEY POINTS

- Clinicians must be aware of most recent literature regarding ortho-biologics and understand the indications for these products in order to inform patients, guide clinical decisions, and manage expectations.
- The process of preparing and delivering the final product can be lengthy and resource intensive, and this must be considered before implementing ortho-biologics into clinical practice.
- To administer ortho-biologics for patients, physicians must familiarize themselves with federal regulations and billing and coding policies of these therapies.
- Perhaps the most important component of incorporating ortho-biologics into clinical practice is to be able to discuss the risks, benefits, alternatives, and expected outcomes of a particular product with patients.

INTRODUCTION

The first and most important step to incorporating ortho-biologics into a clinical practice is to understand the indications for these products. Clinicians must be aware of most recent literature regarding ortho-biologics in order to inform patients, make clinical decisions, and manage expectations. The efficacy of different ortho-biologic

---

Disclosure Statement: See last page of article.
a Center for Orthopaedic Outcomes Research, The Steadman Philippon Research Institute, Vail, CO, USA; b School of Medicine, Oregon Health & Science University, Portland, OR, USA; c The Steadman Clinic, 181 West Meadow Drive Suite 400, Vail, CO 81657, USA
1 Present address: 207 North Roscoe Boulevard, Ponte Verde Beach, FL 32082.
2 Present address: 3601 Southwest River Parkway #2002, Portland, OR 97239.
3 Present address: 181 West Meadow Drive Suite 400, Vail, CO 81657.
* Corresponding author. The Steadman Clinic, Steadman Philippon Research Institute, 181 West Meadow Drive Suite 400, Vail, CO 81657.
E-mail address: mprovencher@thesteadmanclinic.com

therapies has been discussed in detail previously in this issue, but it is important to emphasize that different biologics are used for different pathologies/injuries and in different settings, such as the operating room or in the office.

REGULATIONS, BILLING, AND CODING

To administer ortho-biologics for patients, physicians must familiarize themselves with federal regulations and billing and coding policies of these therapies. The US Food and Drug Administration (FDA) classifies platelet-rich plasma (PRP) as minimally manipulated tissue.[1] Concentrated autologous mesenchymal stem cells (MSCs) do not require FDA approval; however, no products using engineered or expanded MSCs have been approved by the FDA for orthopedic applications.[2] Demineralized bone matrix, which is processed allograft bone, is considered minimally processed tissue and does not require FDA approval.[2]

Insurance companies define biologics as "interventions using cells and biomaterials to support healing and repair."[2] The cost of a single treatment is variable and depends on a variety of factors, including the clinical setting in which the treatment is administered (ie, office vs operating room), need for associated analgesia and/or sedation, and utilization of concomitant image guidance, such as ultrasound or fluoroscopy, among other factors.[3] Many of these interventions, including MSCs, allograft bone products containing viable stem cells, and allograft (**Fig. 1**) or synthetic bone graft substitutes that must be combined with autologous blood or bone marrow, are considered experimental by insurance companies and are, therefore, difficult to obtain approval of coverage.[2] However, many insurance companies are willing to cover biologics that are furnished incident to a physician's treatment,[4] so bundling the cost with surgical procedures, as is performed in the authors' practice, is one way that these therapies may be covered.

The coding requirements of ortho-biologics are constantly evolving, and it is important for physicians to stay up to date on these trends in order to properly code these interventions for billing and insurance purposes. As described throughout the other articles, there is a variety of types of ortho-biologics available; within each category of ortho-biologics, there are multiple different products. This variety makes the specific terminology used in the supporting documentation or procedure note critical to the coding and reimbursement process.[5] As stated previously, ortho-biologics can be administered as an adjuvant in surgery or as a stand-alone procedure in the office setting. If performing an injection during a

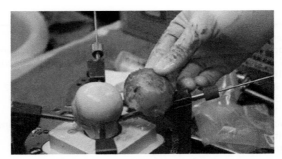

Fig. 1. The resected native humeral head is compared with the fresh osteochondral proximal humeral head allograft. (*Adapted from* Streit JJ, Idoine J, Shishani Y, et al. Operat Tech Sports Med 2015:23(1);24–31. © 2015; with permission.)

surgical procedure, no additional professional service *Current Procedural Terminology (CPT)* coding is reported.[3,5] Coding is required if administered in the office as a stand-alone procedure, and many ortho-biologics have been recognized by *CPT*. PRP, for example, is *0232T: Injections, Platelet Rich Plasma*, which is an all-inclusive code and does not require reporting for the harvesting, spinning, inserting, or radiologic guidance.[5] Despite codes being available, obtaining insurance coverage approval remains difficult. Creative coding, whereby a code that is similar to but does not truly represent a procedure, is not encouraged and can cause difficulties should a provider audit occur.[5]

PREPARATION

Physicians should also be aware of the steps required to harvest and/or prepare ortho-biologics before implementing them into practice. Most of these therapies are harvested from patients, commonly via a peripheral blood draw, bone marrow aspiration, or adipose aspiration. The last two harvest techniques may be performed with patients awake using local analgesia, with sedation, or under general anesthesia (ie, in the operating room). The autologous product is then prepared through some kind of further manipulation, including centrifuge or mixing with other components. The final product is then injected back into patients. PRP, for example, is produced from centrifugation of peripheral blood, a process that concentrates platelets within autologous plasma (**Fig. 2**).[6] After preparation of the harvest site with antiseptic solution, peripheral intravenous access is established and the necessary amount of blood for the procedure (typically 60 mL) is drawn from a peripheral vein in the arm.[6] The blood is then centrifuged per the recommendations of the manufacturer being used. In the senior author's practice, the peripheral blood is spun in the centrifuge at 2600 rotations per minute for 10 minutes, followed by extraction of the top fraction of platelet-poor plasma (PPP), then another 3400 rotations per minute for 6 minutes.[6] Activated PRP preparation is performed by then adding 2 increments of 1.5 mL of PPP and 2 increments of 4.0 mL of diluted PRP.[6] The delivery of PRP for various musculoskeletal conditions can be performed simply by a blind injection, with localization using radiographs or ultrasound, or under direct visualization using fluoroscopy.[6] The process of drawing, preparing, and then injecting the final product can be lengthy and resource intensive; the time, room space, equipment, and personnel required must be considered before implementing ortho-biologics into clinical practice.

PATIENT DISCUSSION

As previously mentioned in this article, perhaps the most important component of incorporating ortho-biologics into clinical practice is to be able to discuss the risks, benefits, alternatives, and expected outcomes of a particular product with patients. This informed consent process is vital to maintaining trust and transparency with patients.[7] Because many ortho-biologics are prepared from autologous blood, there are minimal risks for disease transmission, immunogenic reactions, or cancer.[3] The most common adverse event is donor site morbidity, particularly via the bone marrow aspirate concentrate technique (**Fig. 3**).[4] Less common adverse events include injection site morbidity, infection, or neurovascular injury.[3] The potential benefits from specific ortho-biologics in treating certain musculoskeletal pathologies have been detailed in previous articles. It is important for clinicians to be honest with patients about the most current literature discussing ortho-biologics and to manage their expectations

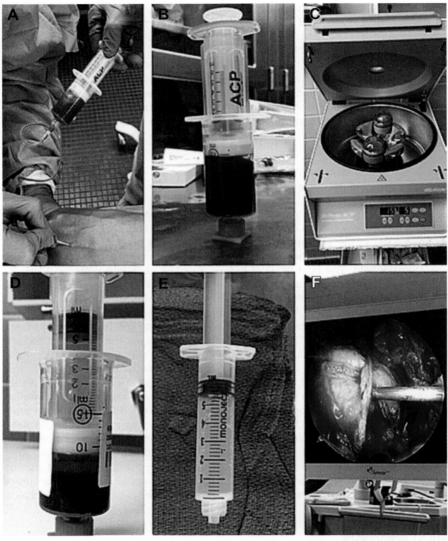

Fig. 2. (*A*) Blood draw in the forearm. (*B*) Final draw of 15 mL of blood. (*C*) Centrifugation at 5000 rotations per minute for 15 minutes. (*D*) Supernatant layer of PRP (*top*) and packed red blood cells (*bottom*). (*E*) Extraction of only supernatant layer of PRP. (*F*) Injection into RCR repair site. RCR, rotator cuff repair. (*Adapted from* Gowd AK, Cabarcas BC, Frank RM, et al. Operat Tech Sports Med 2018:26(1):48–57. © 2018; with permission.)

when receiving these interventions. Much of the current literature is complicated by a lack of standardization of study protocols, harvest and preparation techniques, and outcome measures.[7,8] When treating athletes, it is also important to consider and discuss sporting regulations. It has now generally been agreed by the sporting regulation bodies that the use of autologous blood injections for therapeutic purposes only does not violate the spirit of sport; however, the World Anti-Doping Agency continues to review biologic usage in the light of new scientific information as it becomes

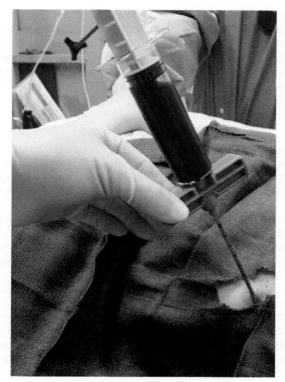

Fig. 3. Bone marrow aspirate is taken from the iliac crest with the use of a needle. The bone marrow aspirate is then processed and concentrated to form an injection solution containing MSCs. (*Adapted from* Lin KM, Wang D, Dines JS. Orthop Clin North Am 2018:49(2):231–9. © 2017; with permission.)

available. Physicians should be aware of any changes in these policies that could jeopardize their patients' playing eligibility.[3]

SUMMARY

The decision to incorporate ortho-biologics into a clinical practice will ultimately depend on physicians' preferences and the resources available to their practice. Physicians thinking about using biologics in their practices should consider the time commitment required to learn and use the technique, insurance coverage, and informed consent.[3] The decision to treat patients with ortho-biologics should be a shared decision based on current literature, previous treatment regimen, and patient goals.

DISCLOSURE STATEMENT

The authors C.P. Murphy, A. Sanchez, and L.A. Peebles have nothing to disclose. M.T. Provencher: AAOS: board or committee member; American Orthopedic Society for Sports Medicine: board or committee member; American Shoulder and Elbow Surgeons: board or committee member; Arthrex, Inc: intellectual property royalties, paid consultant; *Arthroscopy*: editorial or governing board; Arthroscopy Association of North America: board or committee member; International Society of Arthroscopy, Knee Surgery, and Orthopedic Sports Medicine: board or committee member; Joint Restoration Foundation (Allosource): paid consultant; *Knee*: editorial or governing board; *Orthopedics*: editorial or governing board; San Diego Shoulder Institute: board or committee member; SLACK Incorporated: editorial or governing board, publishing royalties, financial or material support; Society of Military Orthopaedic Surgeons: board or committee member.

REFERENCES

1. Chahla J, Cinque ME, Piuzzi NS, et al. A call for standardization in platelet-rich plasma preparation protocols and composition reporting: a systematic review of the clinical orthopaedic literature. J Bone Joint Surg Am 2017;99(20):1769–79.
2. BCBS. Orthopedic applications of stem cell therapy. Corporate medical policy. 2017.
3. Dhillon RS, Schwarz EM, Maloney MD. Platelet-rich plasma therapy - future or trend? Arthritis Res Ther 2012;14(4):219.
4. Medicare. Covered medical and other health services. Medicare benefit policy manual. 2017. Available at: https://www.cms.gov/Regulations-andGuidance/Guidance/Manuals/downloads/bp102c15.pdf.
5. Vaught M, Cole B. Coding and reimbursement issues for platelet-rich plasma. Oper Tech Sports Med 2011;19(1):185–9.
6. Mannava S, Chahla J, Geeslin AG, et al. Platelet-rich plasma augmentation for hip arthroscopy. Arthrosc Tech 2017;6(3):e763–8.
7. Obremskey WT, Marotta JS, Yaszemski MJ, et al. Symposium. The introduction of biologics in orthopaedics: issues of cost, commercialism, and ethics. J Bone Joint Surg Am 2007;89(7):1641–9.
8. Sheth U, Simunovic N, Klein G, et al. Efficacy of autologous platelet-rich plasma use for orthopaedic indications: a meta-analysis. J Bone Joint Surg Am 2012;94(4):298–307.

Moving?

Make sure your subscription moves with you!

To notify us of your new address, find your **Clinics Account Number** (located on your mailing label above your name), and contact customer service at:

Email: journalscustomerservice-usa@elsevier.com

800-654-2452 (subscribers in the U.S. & Canada)
314-447-8871 (subscribers outside of the U.S. & Canada)

Fax number: 314-447-8029

Elsevier Health Sciences Division
Subscription Customer Service
3251 Riverport Lane
Maryland Heights, MO 63043

*To ensure uninterrupted delivery of your subscription, please notify us at least 4 weeks in advance of move.

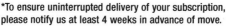

Moving?

Make sure your subscription moves with you!

To notify us of your new address, find your Clinics Account Number (located on your mailing label above your name), and contact customer service at:

Email: journalscustomerservice-usa@elsevier.com

800-654-2452 (subscribers in the U.S. & Canada)
314-447-8871 (subscribers outside of the U.S. & Canada)

Fax number: 314-447-8029

Elsevier Health Sciences Division
Subscription Customer Service
3251 Riverport Lane
Maryland Heights, MO 63043

Printed and bound by CPI Group (UK) Ltd, Croydon, CR0 4YY

08/05/2025

01864741-0002